Neuroanaesthesia: Anaesthesia in a Nutshell

Commissioning editor: Melanie Tait
Development editor: Zoë A. Youd
Production controller: Chris Jarvis
Desk editor: Claire Hutchins
Cover designer: Alan Studholme

Neuroanaesthesia: Anaesthesia in a Nutshell

Judith Dinsmore MBBS FRCA

Consultant Anaesthetist, St George's Hospital and Atkinson Morley's Hospital, London

George Hall MB BS PhD FIBiol FRCA

Professor of Anaesthesia, St George's Hospital and Atkinson Morley's Hospital, London

Series Editors: **Neville Robinson and George Hall**

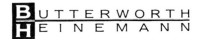

OXFORD AUCKLAND BOSTON JOHANNESBURG MELBOURNE NEW DELHI

Butterworth-Heinemann
Linacre House, Jordan Hill, Oxford OX2 8DP
225 Wildwood Avenue, Woburn, MA 01801-2041
A division of Reed Educational and Professional Publishing Ltd

-℞ A member of the Reed Elsevier plc group

First published 2002

© Reed Educational and Professional Publishing Ltd 2002

British Library Cataloguing in Publication Data
A catalogue record for this book is available from the British Library

Library of Congress Cataloguing in Publication Data
A catalogue record for this book is available from the Library of Congress

ISBN 0 7506 5009 5

For information on all Butterworth-Heinemann
publications please visit our website at www.bh.com

Transferred to digital printing in 2006.

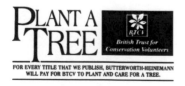

FOR EVERY TITLE THAT WE PUBLISH, BUTTERWORTH-HEINEMANN
WILL PAY FOR BTCV TO PLANT AND CARE FOR A TREE.

Contents

Series preface

Specialist registrars and senior house officers in anaesthesia are now trained by the use of modular educational programmes. In these short periods of intense training the anaesthetist must acquire a fundamental understanding of each anaesthetic specialty. To meet these needs, the trainee requires a concise, pocket-sized book that contains the core knowledge of each subject.

The aims of these nutshell guides are two-fold: first, to provide trainees with the fundamental information necessary for the understanding and safe practice of anaesthesia in each specialty; and secondly, to cover all the key areas of the fellowship examination of the Royal College of Anaesthetists and so act as revision guides for trainees.

P. N. Robinson
G. M. Hall

Preface

Neuroanaesthesia is a challenging subspecialty, and may initially seem daunting to the trainee. It is reassuring to know that despite advances in neuroanaesthesia and the consequent increasing demands and challenges, the fundamental principles remain the same.

There are many excellent large textbooks of neuroanaesthesia. It is not our aim to replace any of these, but rather to produce a pocket-sized guide to the subject whilst still providing a comprehensive source of practical and clinical information for trainees – a book that can be carried around and referred to, both for management problems in theatre and on the neurointensive care unit. In addition, it is hoped that it will provide a useful reference when it comes to revising for the fellowship examination of the Royal College of Anaesthetists.

The topics follow the recommendations of training requirements made by the Neuroanaesthesia Society and the Royal College of Anaesthetists. We hope that this book will fulfil these aims.

Judith Dinsmore
George Hall

List of boxes

Applied neurophysiology

Although many aspects of neuroanaesthesia are common to the practice of anaesthesia as a whole, there are specific problems and clinical situations that are unique to this field. The ability to provide safe anaesthesia and appropriate operating conditions in these circumstances is dependent on a knowledge and understanding of neurophysiology and neuropharmacology.

Cerebral blood flow

The cerebral blood flow (CBF) is derived from the two internal carotid arteries and the two vertebral arteries. The two vertebral arteries join together to form the basilar artery, and this comes together with the internal carotid arteries in the Circle of Willis (Figure 1.1). Venous drainage of the brain is via the venous sinuses, which drain into the internal jugular veins. The cerebral circulation receives 15 per cent of cardiac output, or about 750 ml/min. The mean resting CBF is 50 ml/100 g per min, and this remains remarkably constant under physiological conditions.

The blood–brain barrier

Unlike other capillaries those of the brain are sealed with interendothelial tight junctions, making them relatively impermeable to most substances. This is known as the blood–brain barrier (BBB). Passage through the BBB is determined by lipid solubility, but several hydrophilic substances (including glucose) cross via an active transport system. Permeability increases if the BBB is disrupted, for example following cerebral ischaemia or in acute hypertension. The circumventricular organs (the neurohypophysis and chemoreceptor zones) lie outside the BBB.

Cerebral perfusion

The effective pressure of blood perfusing the brain is the difference between the inflow pressure, taken as the mean arterial entrance pressure at the level of the brain, and the mean venous outflow

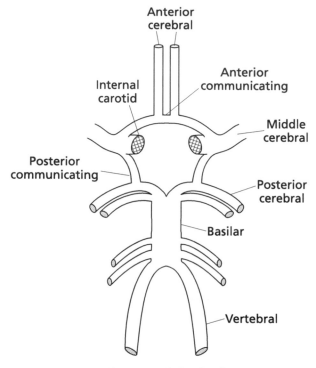

Figure 1.1 Circle of Willis

Box 1.1. Cerebral blood flow

Cerebral blood flow (CBF) accounts for approximately 15 per cent of the cardiac output.

- Resting CBF is 50 ml/100 g min
- Critical CBF is 20 ml/100 g/min.

Cerebral perfusion pressure (CPP) is the difference between mean arterial pressure (MAP) and intracranial pressure (ICP): CPP = MAP − ICP

- Normal CPP is 80 mmHg
- Critical CPP is 40 mmHg.

---

pressure. In practice, the cerebral perfusion pressure (CPP) is taken as the mean arterial pressure (MAP) minus the intracranial pressure (ICP).

$$CPP = MAP - ICP$$

The normal CPP is about 80 mmHg, but this may be reduced if either the MAP falls or the ICP rises.

Control of cerebral blood flow

Autoregulation

Autoregulation is the ability of the cerebral vasculature to maintain a relatively constant blood flow over a range of cerebral perfusion pressures. This is achieved by appropriate alterations in the diameter of the cerebral resistance vessels (CVR), the mechanism of which is unknown but thought to be principally myogenic in origin. The normal range of autoregulation is from 60–150 mmHg. When CPP falls below 60 mmHg, autoregulation fails and CBF decreases; when CPP is greater than 150 mmHg, CBF increases (Figure 1.2). However, the autoregulatory curve may differ between individuals and is modulated by various factors, such as chronic hypertension, when the autoregulatory range is reduced and the curve is shifted to the right. Sympathetic stimulation associated with haemorrhage also moves the curve to the right. Autoregulation is very sensitive to injury in areas of the brain surrounding tumours or abscesses, and autoregulation is lost

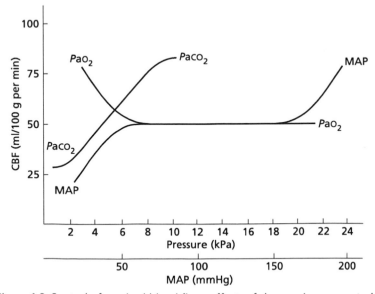

Figure 1.2 Control of cerebral blood flow: effects of changes in mean arterial pressure, $PaCO_2$ and PO_2.

following subarachnoid haemorrhage or head injury. When this happens, CBF becomes dependent on CPP.

Flow–metabolism coupling
Under normal physiological circumstances, total CBF is relatively constant. However, regional differences in CBF occur that parallel neuronal activity in these areas and their increased oxygen consumption (cerebral metabolic rate for oxygen consumption, $CMRO_2$). This coupling between flow and metabolism has been known about for many years, but its exact mechanism is still uncertain. Changes in blood flow occur almost immediately, and suggested mediators include adenosine, K^+, or nitric oxide. This flow–metabolism coupling becomes impaired as a result of a wide variety of interventions, such as anaesthetic drugs and hyperthermia, or cerebral pathology, such as traumatic brain injury.

Carbon dioxide
Carbon dioxide is a potent regulator of CBF. As $PaCO_2$ rises, the cerebral vessels vasodilate and CBF increases; when $PaCO_2$ decreases, CBF falls (Figure 1.2). Within the range 3–10 kPa the relationship between $PaCO_2$ and CBF is linear, with an upper limit of maximal vasodilatation. When $PaCO_2$ falls below 3 kPa, CBF continues to decrease but not so markedly. Carbon dioxide diffuses across the BBB and changes in $PaCO_2$ will be paralleled by changes in the CSF hydrogen ion concentration (H^+). Changes in CBF occurring as a result of changes in $PaCO_2$ are therefore of limited duration, as the changes in (H^+) are buffered by bicarbonate. CBF will have returned to baseline within 6–12 hours.

There is evidence that hyperventilation in intracranial hypertension will become ineffective over a matter of hours due to this adaptive process, but that it also may result in a rebound hyperaemia on return to normocapnoea. An additional problem with hyperventilation is the possibility of a left shift of the oxygen–haemoglobin dissociation curve, reducing the availability of oxygen.

Cerebral reactivity to $PaCO_2$ is impaired in hypotension, head injury and subarachnoid haemorrhage.

Oxygen
The oxygen content of blood rather than the $PaCO_2$ regulates CBF. CBF remains constant as $PaCO_2$ falls until about 6 kPa, when

---

Box 1.2. Control of cerebral blood flow

Flow–metabolism coupling: Regional blood flow alters ∞ activity of the tissue.
Autoregulation, carbon dioxide and oxygen: see Figure 1.2.

---

vasodilatation and a marked increase in CBF occurs (Figure 1.2). CBF doubles as a PaO_2 of 3 kPa is reached. There is little response to increasing PaO_2, with only a 12 per cent reduction in CBF at 1 atmosphere (101 kPa), but this effect does not appear to be clinically significant. Hypoxia impairs autoregulation.

Intracranial pressure

Intracranial contents

Changes in the intracranial pressure (ICP) reflect changes in the volume of the intracranial contents, which consist of brain, cerebrospinal fluid (CSF) and blood:

- Blood volume, 5–10 per cent
- Cerebrospinal fluid (CSF), 10 per cent
- Brain tissue, 80–85 per cent.

The cranium is a fixed, rigid box, and therefore any changes in the contents of this box will vary the pressure within it. In the 1850s the Munro–Kellie hypothesis stated that the contents of the cranium were incompressible and that therefore any increase in intracranial volume would result in a rapid increase in intracranial pressure i.e. the pressure–volume relationship was a straight line. However, this did not take into account either the presence of CSF or the ability to compensate for small changes in volume of one of the contents by decreasing the volume of the other contents.

Blood volume

Although each of the intracranial contents can change in volume, changes in blood volume occur more rapidly than changes in CSF and brain volume. The factors influencing intracranial blood flow have been discussed already. Cerebral vasodilatation is produced by increases in $PaCO_2$ and also occurs with increases in MAP, when autoregulation is impaired. The majority of the intracranial blood volume is contained within the venous system, and this is one of the mechanisms available to compensate for increases in the volume of the other intracerebral contents. There are no valves between the venous sinuses and the superior vena cava; hence if intracranial pressure rises, the capacitance of the cerebral veins decreases and blood is transferred back into the superior vena cava. Conversely, this also means that obstruction of venous drainage will remove this compensatory mechanism and lead to venous congestion, itself causing an increase in ICP. Increases in central venous pressure may be due to straining, coughing or poor positioning of the head and neck. Venous congestion also results in cerebral oedema, which will aggravate any rise in ICP.

Cerebrospinal fluid
Cerebrospinal fluid is produced in the choroid plexus of the lateral ventricles at a rate of 0.3–0.5 ml/min. It flows from here to the third ventricle, via the aqueduct of Sylvius to the fourth ventricle, and enters the subarachnoid space via the foramina of Luschka and Magendie. It is reabsorbed by arachnoid villi into the sagittal sinus by a pressure-dependent process; if venous pressure is raised, CSF reabsorption is slowed. However, normally production balances reabsorption. The total volume of CSF is about 150 ml, and this is equally divided between the cerebral and spinal spaces. The principal function of the CSF is to act as a cushion for the CNS against sudden movements. It also acts as a compensatory mechanism for increases in intracranial volume by displacement of CSF to the spinal subarachnoid space and increased absorption of CSF. Any obstruction to CSF flow, such as aqueduct blockage following subarachnoid haemorrhage or head injury, or any mass that impairs CSF flow, produces hydrocephalus and may result in increased ICP.

Brain
The brain makes up 80–85 per cent of the intracranial contents, and hence any change in its volume will be reflected by a change in ICP. It is a soft and highly compressible organ, but is relatively protected within the confines of the skull and is cushioned by the CSF. These properties mean that a small increase in brain volume, such as a slowly expanding mass lesion, may be accommodated before ICP rises. This usually occurs by a decrease in the capacitance of the intracranial vessels, displacement of CSF into the spinal canal, and then displacement of the brain itself as it occupies this additional space. However, any deformation produced in the process may

result in neurological signs (e.g. midline shift or cranial nerve lesions).

The size and site of an expanding lesion and the speed of expansion will influence the ability to compensate and the neurological signs that develop. There is less room in the posterior fossa, and so signs are seen more quickly. An acute cerebral haematoma allows little time for compensatory mechanisms when compared with a slowly expanding tumour. Some small mass lesions will produce early signs due to associated cerebral oedema.

Cerebral oedema results in a generalized increase in brain volume, and may arise as a result of two mechanisms. Vasogenic oedema is caused by a disruption of the blood–brain barrier, and is characterized by an increase in extracellular fluid. This may be associated with abscesses, neoplasms, trauma or hypertension. In cytotoxic oedema, there is accumulation of intracellular water and sodium due to failure of the cell membrane. It is usually due to hypoxia, and the effects are therefore widespread.

If brain volume continues to increase, compensatory mechanisms fail and the slightest increase in volume, for example due to temporary cerebral vasodilatation, can produce a marked rise in ICP. If intracranial contents are distorted still further, the results can be catastrophic. Supratentorial pressure can cause herniation of the temporal uncus and compression of the brainstem on the contralateral side. This results in an ipsilateral third cranial nerve palsy, decerebrate rigidity, hypertension and bradycardia. Further increases in pressure may result in herniation of the cerebellar tonsils through the foramen magnum and death.

Intracranial pressure

Normal intracranial pressure is 10–15 mmHg, but it is not a static pressure and varies with position, respiration, arterial pulsation, straining etc. There is a limited ability to compensate for increases in volume of intracranial contents before the ICP begins to increase. Slow changes are tolerated better than acute insults. Cerebral compliance is the change in volume per unit change in pressure. When compensatory mechanisms are exhausted the intracranial compliance is greatly reduced and there will be rapid changes in intracranial pressure (ICP). The intracranial pressure–volume relationship is shown in Figure 1.3. A sustained increase in ICP of >15 mmHg is termed intracranial hypertension. However, a raised ICP in isolation, with no local mass effects, will produce few symptoms until a

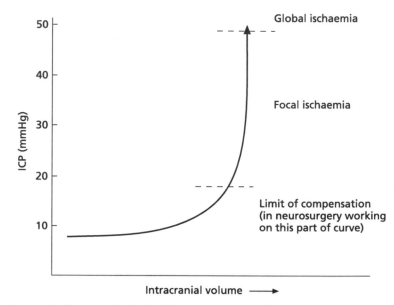

Figure 1.3 There is a limited ability to compensate for increases in intracranial volume (the flat part of the curve). However, when these mechanisms are exhausted, small volume increases can produce marked rises in ICP.

critical point is reached. At this point cerebral perfusion is reduced to the point when cerebral ischaemia occurs. The cerebral perfusion pressure (CPP) is dependent on the difference between the mean arterial pressure (MAP) and the intracranial pressure (ICP):

$$CPP = MAP - ICP$$

CBF is autoregulated and CBF is maintained despite changing blood pressure (within MAP 60–160 mmHg), but as ICP rises this ability is lost. If ICP is greater than 20 mmHg, areas of focal ischaemia appear; at ICP greater than 50 mmHg, global ischaemia occurs. CPP is an important therapeutic target in the management of raised ICP.

Raised ICP occurs in neurosurgical patients as a result of an increase in cerebral blood volume (e.g. haematoma, hyperaemia), an increase in volume of CSF (e.g. hydrocephalus), or an increased volume of brain tissue (e.g. tumour or cerebral oedema). The significance of a raised ICP is two-fold:

1. It will decrease cerebral perfusion
2. It will cause distortion and displacement of cerebral contents.

Box 1.3. Intracranial pressure

The skull is of fixed volume, so a change in volume of any of the intracranial contents will result in changes in *intracranial pressure* (ICP). The intracranial contents are:

- Cerebral blood volume, 5–10 per cent
- Cerebrospinal fluid, 10 per cent
- Brain tissue, 80–85 per cent (60 per cent water, 40 per cent solid).

The relationship between intracranial pressure and volume is shown in Figure 1.3.
The normal ICP is 10–15 mmHg.

Measurement of ICP

Diagnosis of a raised ICP solely on clinical signs is often unreliable, as is diagnosis based on a solitary reading such as lumbar puncture (LP). The gold standard for measuring ICP remains the intraventricular catheter; alternative methods are discussed in Chapter 9. Measurement of ICP and analysis of the trace provide useful information, not just about the actual ICP but also giving an indication of disease progression and the response to treatment. The normal ICP trace has pulsations corresponding to the heart rate, and slower waves reflecting respiration. With increasing ICP abnormal waves appear, as first described by Lundberg in 1960 (Continuous recording and control of ventricular fluid pressure in neurosurgical practice. *Acta Psychiatrica et Neurologica Scandinavica* **36** (Suppl. 149), 81–176). A waves or plateau waves indicate large rises in ICP (up to 80 mmHg) that may persist for up to 20 minutes. During this time the CPP falls, leading to vasodilatation and a further rise in ICP. These waves occur in patients approaching the limits of compensation. B waves are smaller than A waves (up to 25 mmHg) and of shorter duration (0.5–2 minutes). They may precede the development of A waves. C waves are of limited duration and amplitude.

2

Applied neuropharmacology

Recent developments in neuroanaesthesia are due in part to the availability of new anaesthetic agents. However, operative conditions depend on many inter-related factors and anaesthetic agents play only a small role; hence the need to have an understanding of both cerebral neurophysiology and neuropharmacology.

Ideally agents used in neuroanaesthesia should not increase cerebral blood flow, decrease cerebral autoregulation or impair cerebral reactivity to carbon dioxide. In addition, anaesthetic agents should permit rapid changes in the depth of anaesthesia intraoperatively and allow rapid recovery on completion of surgery.

Effects of drugs on cerebral blood flow and intracranial pressure
Volatile agents
All volatile anaesthetic agents alter cerebral blood flow (CBF). This happens both by a direct effect on vascular smooth muscle and indirectly by their effect on cerebral metabolic rate (CMR). The CMR is reduced – by differing amounts – by all agents, and in decreasing metabolism this reduces CBF. Halothane reduces CMR less than isoflurane at equipotent concentrations. However, this difference becomes less marked if global, as opposed to regional, CMR is studied, as isoflurane produces greater cortical metabolic suppression. As the concentration of volatile agent is increased, vasodilatation will occur with marked increases in CBF. These increases are less with isoflurane at concentrations used in anaesthesia, and at present it is the volatile agent most often used for neuroanaesthesia. Carbon dioxide reactivity appears to be retained during administration of isoflurane, and isoflurane confers better cerebral protection than halothane and enflurane. However sevoflurane may have some advantages; it causes less vasodilatation than isoflurane at equipotent concentrations. At 1.5 MAC (minimal alveolar concentration) it does not increase CBF and preserves autoregulation and CO_2 reactivity. The

⎯rovascular effects of desflurane seem to be very similar to those of isoflurane. Since the discovery that enflurane may produce epileptiform activity it is no longer used in neuroanaesthesia.

Volatile agents may increase ICP, especially when intracranial compliance is reduced. This effect is probably a result of changes in CBF, but is modified by the underlying physiological conditions. Hypoventilation, with an increasing $PaCO_2$, will cause a further increase in CBF, which will obviously increase ICP – perhaps dangerously. Conversely, increases in ICP associated with these agents may be attenuated by prior hyperventilation. There have been reports of both desflurane and sevoflurane producing greater rises in ICP than does isoflurane.

Nitrous oxide

Nitrous oxide produces cerebrovasodilatation and a decrease in autoregulatory capacity. At equipotent MAC values its effects are more marked than those of halothane and isoflurane. Nitrous oxide has also been shown to increase CMR. Nitrous oxide increases ICP in patients with reduced cerebral compliance.

Intravenous agents

The intravenous agents thiopentone, etomidate and propofol all decrease CMR and $CMRO_2$. This reduction in $CMRO_2$ is proportional to the depth of anaesthesia and continues until electrical activity is abolished, producing an isoelectric EEG. These intravenous agents also produce marked and dose-dependent decreases in CBF, partly as a consequence of the depression of cerebral function. There is no effect on autoregulation and CO_2 reactivity. Benzodiazepines reduce CMR and CBF, but the effect is less pronounced than with propofol or thiopentone.

As a consequence of these effects on CMR and CBF, propofol and thiopentone both decrease ICP. Indeed they have been used both on the neurosurgical intensive care unit and during operative procedures to control ICP. Propofol is particularly useful in neuroanaesthesia. Its pharmacological profile, high metabolic clearance, rapid elimination and linear pharmacokinetics allow it to be given by infusion, whilst still providing good recovery characteristics. Initial worries about its effects on cerebral perfusion secondary to decreases in mean arterial pressure (MAP) have proved unfounded. Etomidate produces similar effects to propofol and thiopentone on cerebral haemodynamics and ICP. In addition, it produces little cardiovascular depression, even in the high-risk individual. However, it has fallen out of favour because it suppresses adrenocortical function. Benzodiazepines have little effect on ICP. The exception to the above is ketamine, which increases CMR and CBF. Ketamine also increases ICP, and, although these changes may be partially attenuated by hypocapnia or other intravenous agents, ketamine is avoided in patients with decreased intracranial compliance. However, there has been some renewed interest recently because of its antagonist effect at the NMDA receptor and, hence, potential cerebroprotective effect.

Neuromuscular blocking drugs
Non-depolarizing muscle relaxants do not cross the blood–brain barrier (BBB) and have little effect on CMR or CBF and hence on ICP. Suxamethonium is associated with a rise in ICP as a consequence of muscle fasciculation and hypertension. These changes are transient, and may be attenuated by adequate doses of induction agent or pre-dosing with a small dose of non-depolarizing relaxant. Securing the airway, and avoiding hypoxia and hypercapnia take priority, and suxamethonium should be used if indicated.

Opioids
Opiates seem to have little effect on CBF or on autoregulation at clinically relevant doses. Large doses of fentanyl, sufentanil and remifentanil depress CMR and hence decrease CBF, but often also decrease MAP at these doses. Remifentanil seems ideally suited to neuroanaesthesia. It is a μ-receptor agonist, which is rapidly metabolized by plasma and tissue esterases. It has a context sensitive half-life of about 2 minutes, and can be given by infusion without accumulation. It provides haemodynamic stability and a rapid recovery. Postoperative analgesia may be a problem, and alternative analgesia should be instituted early to avoid hypertension during the recovery period.

The effects of anaesthetic agents on cerebral haemodynamics are summarized in Box 2.1.

Adjuvant drugs
Increases in blood pressure may occur at various stages during neurosurgical procedures, and are most commonly associated with laryngoscopy, intubation and painful stimuli. Whilst extreme hypertension should be avoided, it is equally important to avoid

---

Box 2.1. The effects of anaesthetic agents on cerebral haemodynamics

	CBF	CMRO$_2$	Autoregulation	ICP	CSF production
Volatile agents					
Halothane	↑	↓	impaired	↑	↔
Enflurane	↑	↓	impaired	↑	↔
Isoflurane	↑	↓	impaired	↑	↔
Sevoflurane	↑	↓	impaired	↑	↔
Desflurane	↑	↓	impaired	↑	↔
Nitrous oxide	↑	↑	impaired	↑	↔
Intravenous agents					
Propofol	↓	↓	↔	↓	↔
Thiopentone	↓	↓	↔	↓	↔
Etomidate	↓	↓	↔	↓	↓
Midazolam	↓	↓	↔	↓	↔
Ketamine	↑	↑	↔	↑	↔
Neuromuscular blocking drugs					
Non-depolarizing	↔	↔	↔	↔	↔
Suxamethonium	↑	↑	↔	↑	↔
Opioids	↔	↓	↔	↑^{S}	↔
Mannitol	↔	↔	↔	↓	↓

↓, decreased; ↑, increased; ↔, no change; ↑^{S}, increased but short lived.

---

prolonged periods of hypotension. Autoregulation of CBF may be impaired in neurosurgical patients, and increases in MAP in these patients will lead to increases in CBF and ICP. There are various methods of attenuating these hypertensive responses:

- *Opioids* – short-lived, painful stimuli are probably best managed by additional opioids or by increasing the level of anaesthesia.
- *Lignocaine* (1.5 mg/kg) has been used to reduce the haemodynamic response to laryngoscopy. It has been suggested that a bolus dose prior to intubation, decreases ICP without compromising haemodynamic stability.
- *Antihypertensives* – if blood pressure is unacceptably high despite adequate anaesthesia, specific antihypertensive drugs may be needed.

Antihypertensive drugs
1 *Beta-blockers* have become the mainstay of antihypertensive therapy in this setting. Labetalol or esmolol have both been used.

Esmolol is relatively cardioselective and has a very short duration of action; it is useful when large increases in blood pressure need immediate resolution. Labetalol is a mixed alpha and beta-blocker; it has an additional arteriolar vasodilating action and it decreases cardiac output and peripheral vascular resistance. It has no effect on ICP even when intracranial compliance is reduced, and it is given in 2.5–5 mg increments.

2 *Sodium nitroprusside* is also useful. It is given by infusion (maximum dose 1.5 µg/kg per min) and acts on arteriolar tone to reduce cardiac output. It has a rapid onset and offset of action, and the infusion rate can be titrated against blood pressure. Sodium nitroprusside has a variable effect on CBF and ICP, dependent on dosage and rate of administration. It does seem to impair autoregulation. Accumulation of cyanide metabolites resulting in cyanide toxicity is not a problem in the short term.

3 *Hydralazine* is a smooth muscle blocking agent. It increases ICP and impairs autoregulation, but despite this it has been widely used and does not seem to cause problems in clinical practice if given slowly.

4 *Glyceryl trinitrate* dilates the venous capacitance vessels and has a short half-life. It increases CBF and ICP.

5 *Calcium channel blockers* interfere with the inward displacement of calcium ions through the slow channels of active cell membranes. Although many of these drugs are used in the treatment of hypertension, nimodipine is used almost exclusively in neurosurgical patients. It acts preferentially on the vascular smooth muscle of cerebral arteries, and is used for the prevention and treatment of vasospasm following subarachnoid haemorrhage. It has also been shown to have a cerebroprotective effect.

Diuretics

1 *Mannitol* is used to control ICP and reduce cerebral oedema in neurosurgical patients (see also Chapter 4). It is given as intermittent boluses of 0.25 g/kg. Mannitol has a complicated mechanism of action:

• It withdraws water from areas of brain with an intact blood–brain barrier into the intravascular compartment and so reduces brain tissue volume
• It lowers blood haematocrit and hence reduces CBV

- It decreases CSF production
- It is also a free radical scavenger.

However, its high osmolarity means that it produces a temporary hypervolaemia and it should be used with caution in patients with significant cardiac disease, in whom it might precipitate cardiac failure. Renal excretion of mannitol promotes a diuresis, which leads to systemic dehydration, and excessive use may produce hyperosmolality. Mannitol can produce vasodilatation, resulting in a temporarily increased ICP and a drop in MAP. However it seems that this phenomenon does not occur in the presence of intracranial hypertension or when it is given slowly.

2 *Frusemide* is also used to control ICP and reduce brain swelling, although its maximal effect is delayed compared with that of mannitol. Its exact mechanism of action remains uncertain, although it seems to be related to its ability to block chloride transport. Its initial actions are by reducing cell swelling rather than reducing extracellular volume.

Control of convulsions

Seizures are a relatively common occurrence in neurosurgical patients. In addition many high-risk patients are given prophylactic anticonvulsants perioperatively, so the neuroanaesthetist must be familiar with these drugs. The object of treatment is to prevent the occurrence of seizures by maintaining an effective plasma concentration of the appropriate drug (see also Chapter 12). Anticonvulsant drugs have complex drug interactions. As the result of hepatic enzyme induction there may be accelerated recovery from neuromuscular blockade.

1 *Phenytoin* is effective in most types of epilepsy and in status epilepticus. It has a narrow therapeutic index and the relationship between dose and the plasma concentration is non-linear; hence the importance of monitoring plasma concentrations. To achieve effective plasma concentrations a loading dose is required; 15 mg/kg, at a rate of not more than 50 mg/min, followed by maintenance dosage. Side effects of phenytoin are numerous, but in this setting hypotension, dysrhythmias, respiratory depression and even cardiovascular collapse may occur, particularly if given too rapidly.

2 *Phenobarbitone* has the same indications as above. It may be sedative. The dose is 15 mg/kg i.v. at no more than 50 mg/min; intramuscular absorption is effective but slow.

3 *Benzodiazepines.* Benzodiazepines penetrate the brain rapidly and are potent GABA agonists, improving local inhibition of signal transmission. They are used in the immediate management of status epilepticus. Diazepam is the most commonly used; a 10–20 mg i.v. bolus at the rate of 2.5 mg per 30 seconds. This dose can be repeated at 30-minute intervals. It may also be given by intravenous infusion or rectally; intramuscular absorption is unreliable and should be avoided. There is a danger of respiratory depression. Other benzodiazepines used include lorazepam, clonazepam and midazolam.

4 *Chlormethiazole* is useful in status epilepticus. It is given as a 0.8 per cent solution, at 15 ml/min up to 100 ml, and then the rate is reduced to maintain control of seizures. At these doses intubation and ventilation are usually required. The large volumes of fluid used during these infusions may result in volume overload and electrolyte problems.

5 *Anaesthetic agents.* Thiopentone and propofol are both useful in the treatment of status epilepticus. Patients will obviously need ventilation and occasionally inotropic support during infusion. Thiopentone is very lipid-soluble and accumulates on prolonged infusion, leading to delayed recovery. There is less experience with propofol, but it has useful anticonvulsant properties and is rapidly metabolized. Isoflurane has some anticonvulsant properties but it seems to suppress the spread of seizure activity rather than suppress the active focus.

Management of cerebral ischaemia

Neuroprotective agents have been the subject of much research over recent years, as understanding of the pathophysiology of cerebral ischaemia increases. At present, there is still little available pharmacologically to reduce permanent injury from cerebral ischaemia. The most important clinical advance has been the recognition of the importance of manipulation of physiological variables both intraoperatively and in the ITU.

Mechanisms to reduce cerebral metabolic rate

Ischaemia will reduce the supply of metabolic substrates, and therefore drugs that decrease metabolic demand should influence energy balance favourably and prolong tolerance to, or improve outcome, from a temporary ischaemic insult. The classic agent used for this purpose is thiopentone, which reduces CMR by about 50 per cent and is accompanied by depression of the EEG. When the EEG becomes isoelectric no further reduction of CMR can be achieved by additional doses of drug. However, experimental evidence has largely discredited this theory. Although anaesthetic agents do seem to afford some benefit during focal ischaemia, this probably does not result from their ability to reduce CMR, and they do not provide protection against global ischaemia.

Hypothermia

There has been renewed interest in the role of hypothermia over recent years. Attention has focused on mild hypothermia (34–35°C) rather than the profound hypothermia abandoned previously. In experimental models, even cooling the brain by 2–3°C reduced ischaemic injury. Mild hypothermia has also been found to be beneficial in head injury. Clinical trials are still underway regarding its applications and outcomes.

Hyperglycaemia

The association between hyperglycaemia and worsened outcome from global ischaemia has been validated. Hyperglycaemia initiates anaerobic glycolysis and the resultant lactic acidosis leads to deregulation of glucose metabolism, ionic homeostasis, and results in free radical formation. However, there is as yet no evidence that aggressive control of hyperglycaemia with insulin will improve outcome, and hypoglycaemia must be avoided.

Neuroprotective drugs

These agents are still experimental. The following appear promising:

1 Calcium antagonists, which have shown moderate efficacy in stroke but none against global ischaemia
2 Antagonists to excitatory amino acid neurotransmitters:
   • NMDA antagonists – compounds that antagonize glutamate at NMDA receptor have produced dramatic results in focal ischaemia, but again seem ineffective in global ischaemia

- AMPA antagonists – compounds that antagonize glutamate at AMPA receptors have been found to be protective against both focal ischaemia and global ischaemia.

3 Free radical scavengers.

3

Principles of anaesthesia
for craniotomy

Neurosurgical anaesthesia is one branch of the specialty in which close collaboration between the anaesthetist and surgeon is essential. The conduct of the anaesthetic may affect the outcome by control of ICP and brain volume, a decrease in arterial pressure to reduce haemorrhage, and possibly by offering some protection from cerebral ischaemia.

Control of ICP is particularly important in the early stages of surgery; the ICP is atmospheric when the skull is opened. Even when the skull is open, increases in CBF will increase the brain volume. More vigorous retraction is then needed for surgical access with enhanced potential for local ischaemia and post-operative oedema.

Principles of neuroanaesthesia
The principles outlined in Box 3.1 are fundamental, and are much more important than the anaesthetic agents used.

Airway and ventilation
A perfect airway is essential at all times – pre-, intra- and post-operatively – in neurosurgical patients. It is usually ensured during surgery by the use of a flexometallic reinforced tracheal

---

Box 3.1. Principles of neuroanaesthesia

- Perfect airway and controlled ventilation to achieve adequate oxygenation and hypocarbia
- Stable arterial pressure
- Prevention of factors that increase CVP
- Careful i.v. fluid balance
- Avoidance of anaesthetic techniques that increase ICP and use of methods to decrease brain volume.

tube that is fixed sufficiently firmly to withstand all surgical interference! Ventilation to moderate hypocapnia (a $PaCO_2$ of about 4 kPa) is sufficient to cause a decrease in CBF and ICP. More vigorous hyperventilation down to a $PaCO_2$ of 3 kPa is no longer used routinely, as CBF changes little at $PaCO_2 < 3$ kPa. High minute volumes may increase the CVP, and it has been suggested that very low $PaCO_2$ values may be associated with cerebral ischaemia. When moderate hyperventilation is continued for many hours, CBF slowly returns to normal but ICP may remain decreased for longer because of a decline in intracranial CSF volume.

Control of arterial pressure

Major fluctuations in arterial pressure must be prevented in neuroanaesthesia. Hypertension can result in an increase in ICP in patients with impaired or abolished autoregulation and, if persistent, cerebral oedema may ensue. Patients needing surgery for clipping of a cerebral aneurysm or following traumatic brain injury already have increased sympathetic nervous system activity, and hypertension must be prevented. The main stimuli for catecholamine release are:

- Laryngoscopy and intubation
- Insertion of pins
- Raising of bone flap
- Completion of surgery and emergence from anaesthesia.

The main methods of preventing hypertension are:

- Deepening anaesthesia
- Use of opioids
- Use of hypotensive drugs.

Hypotension is less of a problem, and some lowering of arterial pressure is common after induction of anaesthesia and before surgery starts. If severe, there may be a significant decline in cerebral perfusion pressure. On the other hand, mild hypotension seems to reduce brain bulk and is sometimes associated with improved operating conditions.

Prevention of increase in CVP

Increases in CVP must be avoided, as these result in increases in ICP. Simple mechanical factors that raise CVP include:

- Coughing and straining
- Head positions that obstruct the neck veins
- Pressure on abdomen and thorax
- Incorrect position of patient – a 'head-up' position is essential
- Positive end expiratory pressure on ventilation of lungs
- Cannulation of jugular veins.

The transmission of changes in CVP to ICP occurs principally by two routes: first, an increase in CVP is transmitted to the jugular and vertebral veins to raise cerebral venous pressure and hence ICP; and secondly, an increase in pressure in the veins in the epidural space raises CSF pressure. The second route is more important when rapid increases in intrathoracic pressure occur, such as with coughing.

Intravenous fluids
In patients with an intact blood–brain barrier, plasma osmolality rather than the plasma colloid osmotic pressure controls the water flux between the circulation and the brain. For many neurosurgical patients it can be assumed that the function of the blood–brain barrier is impaired.

The crystalloid of choice in neurosurgical patients is 0.9 per cent sodium chloride solution. It is slightly hyperoncotic compared with serum (300 mosm/kg compared with 285 mosm/kg). Hartmann's solution (Ringer's lactate) is not used because it has an osmolality of around only 250 mosm/kg. Hypotonic solutions such as 5 per cent glucose and 4 per cent glucose in 0.18 per cent sodium chloride are contraindicated absolutely, except occasionally in diabetic patients. They raise ICP and increase the risk of cerebral oedema. Furthermore, circulating blood glucose values > 10 mmol/l must be prevented as they increase the likelihood of greater brain damage if cerebral ischaemia occurs.

It is usual to infuse 0.9 per cent sodium chloride i.v. at a sufficient rate to ensure cardiovascular stability and hence cerebral perfusion, but avoid overhydration. Once any preoperative deficits have been corrected, an infusion rate of around 100 ml/h is often adequate.

Colloid solutions are used if cardiovascular stability cannot be maintained with crystalloid infusions. Modified gelatins or hydroxethyl starch are commonly infused after 2 l of crystalloid solutions have been given. Fluid restriction postoperatively is no longer undertaken.

Box 3.2. Techniques to decrease cranial contents

- Removal of CSF   Ventricular drain   Lumbar drain
- Diuretics   Mannitol   Loop diuretics
- Glucocorticoids   Dexamethasone
- Excision of space-occupying lesion Blood
                                     Tumour
                                     Brain

Techniques to decrease cranial contents

It is often necessary to use methods to decrease the volume of the cranial contents to aid surgery (see Box 3.2). This can be achieved by a reduction in one or more of the following:

- Cerebral blood volume
- CSF volume
- Brain tissue.

Removal of CSF

A ventricular drain may be inserted preoperatively and CSF drained to maintain a normal ICP. Lumbar drains are usually inserted after induction of anaesthesia, particularly in patients undergoing posterior fossa surgery and clipping of cerebral aneurysms. Lumbar drains must not be opened before the bone flap is lifted.

Diuretics

Mannitol is commonly used to decrease a raised ICP. Although mannitol is an osmotic diuretic, the initial decline in ICP is independent of the diuresis. An effect on ICP is usually noted within a few minutes, is maximal after 30 minutes, and lasts for up to 2 hours after a typical dose of 0.25–0.5 mg/kg i.v. In addition to its osmotic diuretic properties, mannitol has been shown to decrease cerebrovascular resistance and blood viscosity and so increase flow in ischaemic areas of brain.

Loop diuretics such as frusemide are used in some centres, as they decrease ICP without altering serum osmolality or cerebral blood flow. Occasionally both mannitol and a loop diuretic are given.

Glucocorticoids

Dexamethasone is given preoperatively to decrease cerebral oedema. It has a slow onset of action.

Excision of space-occupying lesion
Evacuation of a haematoma or debulking of a cerebral tumour is often the indication for surgery. Surgical access is improved if the volume of the cranial contents is reduced. Occasionally it is necessary to excise parts of normal brain, either to gain access to the lesion or to close the skull. The frontal or temporal poles are commonly sacrificed.

Preoperative assessment
Evaluation of the patient before surgery is used to assess the anaesthetic risks for the proposed surgery, to decide the anaesthetic technique and to plan postoperative care. An explanation of the relevant details of the anaesthetic is given to the patient, and the use of premedication (if any) discussed. The assessment of the neurosurgical patient is identical to that used in all patients, but special attention must be given to the following:

1 An evaluation of ICP. This may be simple if ICP is measured, for example following TBI (traumatic brain injury), for example, or if there are symptoms and signs such as headache, vomiting and papilloedema. Even if these are absent, the presence of a large space-occupying lesion in the brain indicates decreased intracranial compliance.
2 Effects of the intracranial pathology. It has been suggested that if there is gross oedema around the tumour on the CT scan, then these patients are more likely to develop raised ICP during surgery. Patients with depressed consciousness for several days may have delayed gastric emptying, aspiration pneumonitis and impaired vasomotor tone.
3 Treatment given for the pathology. Unfortunately, there are few specific treatments that have been shown to be of benefit in neurosurgical patients. Patients may be prescribed the following drugs, which should be continued up to, and including, the day of surgery:

- Dexamethasone
- Anticonvulsants
- Nimodipine.

Preoperative investigations of the neurosurgical patient are similar to those for patients undergoing general surgery, but special attention must be given to a recent determination of circulating electrolyte values and a clotting screen. Specific considerations are described in the subsequent chapters.

Basic neuroanaesthetic technique

As for other anaesthetic specialties, there is no single 'correct' list of suitable anaesthetic agents. Some anaesthetists achieve excellent results supplementing anaesthesia with a volatile agent such as isoflurane, while others use a total intravenous technique (TIVA) with a propofol infusion + opioid. High doses of opioids are not necessary, however, because the scalp is usually infiltrated with a local anaesthetic and the surgery is unstimulating after the bone flap has been raised. The following outline describes a typical neuroanaesthetic:

- *Premedication* – Glycopyrrolate i.m.
- *Induction* – Thiopentone or propofol, + opioid (e.g. fentanyl 3 µg/ kg). The aim is to minimize increases in heart rate and blood pressure
- *Neuromuscular blocking drug* – Vecuronium or atracurium, but suxamethonium if rapid sequence induction is indicated. Initially, a large bolus of non-depolarizing blocking drug is given to ensure perfect paralysis at laryngoscopy and intubation, followed by an infusion the rate of which is varied according to assessment with a peripheral nerve stimulator. The lateral popliteal nerve is often used for this purpose
- *After tracheal intubation* – Fix tracheal tube securely
  Tape eyes
  ? Insert urinary catheter
  ? Insert lumbar drain
  ? Insert pharyngeal pack
  Check position of patient (ensure the tracheal tube has not moved).

Hypotension after induction

This is a common occurrence, and is usually due to relative fluid depletion preoperatively and a prolonged period of anaesthesia before surgery. Most patients respond to the rapid infusion of 0.9 per cent sodium chloride solution; vasopressors such as ephedrine are needed occasionally. Raising the legs can be a useful short-term measure, but the Trendelenburg position is absolutely contraindicated.

Box 3.3. Intraoperative monitoring

Cardiovascular system ECG
 Arterial pressure–indirect and direct
 CVP
Respiratory system S_pO_2
 E_tCO_2 .
 F_iO_2
 F_i volatile agent
 Minute volume
 Arterial blood gases (used to calibrate end-tidal CO_2)
Fluids Urine volume
 Circulating electrolytes
 Haemoglobin or haematocrit
Temperature Nasopharyngeal temperature
Neuromuscular blockade Peripheral nerve stimulator

Start of surgery

The surgeon usually infiltrates the scalp with a local anaesthetic + adrenaline, which often results in a small decline in arterial pressure. At this time it is commonplace to give i.v. antibiotics and anticonvulsants.

Maintenance of anaesthesia

Isoflurane supplementation of a N_2O/O_2 mixture is often used. Nitrous oxide is frequently omitted in posterior fossa surgery. The aim is to provide good operating conditions to facilitate surgery. Hypertensive responses may be treated by increasing the inspired concentration of isoflurane (but note the adverse effects on cerebral blood volume at >1.5 MAC isoflurane) by a bolus dose of opioid or increasing opioid infusion or by giving adrenergic blocking drugs such as labetalol. Intraoperative monitoring is summarized in Box 3.3.

Emergence and extubation

The conclusion of surgery is often painful, with the suturing of the scalp, insertion of skin clips and removal of pins. Anaesthesia must be maintained to ensure cardiovascular stability, together with any antihypertensive regimen; the $PaCO_2$ allowed to rise slowly; and neuromuscular blockade reversed when the first twitch of a train-of-four is present. The tracheal tube is removed as soon as possible to reduce the likelihood of coughing.

Surgical problems

These can arise during the conduct of an apparently routine anaesthetic. The operating conditions may be poor with a swollen brain. Surgeons are very quick to recognize this difficulty, and soon ask for help. The following interventions are often useful, but must only be undertaken after the anaesthetic technique has been very carefully checked, *particularly the airway and adequacy of ventilation*:

• Administration of bolus of thiopentone or propofol
• Removal of CSF
• Administration of diuretic, or further dose if already given
• Provision of moderate hypotension
• Hyperventilation down to a $PaCO_2$ of 3 kPa
• Administration of dexamethasone i.v. for effect postoperatively.

If the brain swelling occurs abruptly and is massive, then in addition to a bolus of thiopentone and removal of CSF a partial frontal or temporal lobectomy may be necessary.

Stereotatic procedures

Stereotatic procedures are increasingly being used, often to biopsy lesions in deep or functionally important regions of brain. General anaesthesia may present problems, as access to the airway becomes impossible once the rigid headframe is in position.

Postoperative care

This is discussed fully in Chapter 10. Again, the emphasis should be maintenance of a perfect airway with adequate ventilation. Respiratory problems are the most frequent cause of deterioration in the patient's neurological status.

4

Anaesthesia for aneurysm surgery

It has been stated that 1–2 per cent of the population have an intracranial arterial aneurysm. If so, then it is fortunate that the majority do not rupture. The incidence of subarachnoid haemorrhage (SAH) from aneurysm rupture is about 100 cases per 100 000 population per year. Even with modern neurosurgical management, only about 25–30 per cent of patients with a SAH return to their premorbid state after surgery. SAH is more common in women than men, and the greatest incidence is in the age group 40–60 years.

Aneurysms may present as a subarachnoid haemorrhage (the most common presentation), as a space-occupying lesion or as a cranial nerve palsy, and unruptured aneurysms may be an incidental finding. When an intracranial aneurysm ruptures ICP increases rapidly to approach arterial pressure, resulting in the characteristic severe headache, and consciousness is lost if there is cerebral ischaemia. The increase in ICP is usually transient. A meningeal reaction to the blood occurs, with persistent headache, photophobia, neck stiffness and fever. The intracerebral bleed activates the sympatho-adrenal system and can result in hypertension, cardiac arrhythmias, areas of focal myocardial necrosis, leucocytosis and occasionally neurogenic pulmonary oedema. Many patients also have a persistent hypercortisolaemia.

The severity of SAH can be graded according to one of two main grading scales; the Hunt and Hess scale (Box 4.1) and the World Federation of Neurological Surgeons (WFNS) scale (Box 4.2).

Complications of subarachnoid haemorrhage
Complications are important contributors to mortality and morbidity in the 2 weeks after SAH. The main complications are listed in Box 4.3.

Box 4.1. Hunt and Hess Subarachnoid Haemorrhage (SAH) Scale

Grade	Description
0	Unruptured aneurysm
I	Asymptomatic; or minimal headache and slight neck rigidity
II	Moderate to severe headache, neck rigidity; no neurological deficit or cranial nerve palsy
III	Drowsiness, confusion or mild focal deficit
IV	Stupor; moderate to severe hemiparesis; possibly early decerebrate rigidity
V	Deep coma, decerebrate rigidity; moribund appearance

Note that serious systemic disease such as hypertension, coronary artery disease, chronic pulmonary disease and severe vasospasm on angiography result in the patient being demoted by one category.

Box 4.2. World Federation of Neurological Surgeons (WFNS) SAH Scale

WFNS grade	GCS score	Motor deficit
0	Unruptured aneurysm	
I	15	Absent
II	14–13	Absent
III	14–13	Present
IV	12–7	Present or absent
V	6–3	Present or absent

GCS = Glasgow Coma Scale (see Chapter 9).

Box 4.3. Complications of subarachnoid haemorrhage
- Rebleeding
- Raised ICP
- Decreased CBF
- Fluid and electrolyte disorders
- Catecholamine-mediated changes
- Vasospasm.

Rebleeding

This occurs commonly, in about 20 per cent in the first 2 weeks, and is frequently fatal. The risk is maximal on the first day and diminishes with time. For this reason aneurysms are usually operated on as soon as possible after angiographic confirmation of the diagnosis.

Raised ICP
Intracranial pressure usually returns to normal rapidly after the SAH. However, a secondary rise may occur. The use of ICP monitoring is uncommon, but if acute hydrocephalus occurs then ventricular drainage may be undertaken. Sudden decompression increases the risk of rebleeding.

Decreased CBF
Cerebral blood flow is related to the clinical grade, and is decreased still further in focal areas of vasospasm. Autoregulation and CO_2 reactivity are often impaired in patients with poor clinical grades.

Fluid and electrolyte disorders
There is a decrease in blood volume, probably as a consequence of increased sympathoadrenal activity. Consequently most SAH patients are infused intravenously with 3 l/day 0.9 per cent sodium chloride solution. This i.v. fluid regimen also helps to treat the hyponatraemia that can occur after SAH. The mechanism responsible for this natriuresis – the salt-wasting syndrome of SAH – is currently thought to be increased secretion of brain natriuretic peptide (BNP).

Catecholamine-mediated changes
Excessive sympathetic activity can persist for many days, and the effects include cardiac arrhythmias (ECG changes occur in >50 per cent of patients), myocardial necrosis, hypertension, neurogenic pulmonary oedema and a leucocytosis.

Vasospasm
Vasospasm occurs in about 25 per cent of patients with SAH, commonly 5–10 days after the initial bleed. After rebleeding, the delayed neurological deterioration from spasm is the next biggest contributor to morbidity and mortality following SAH. Spasm involves the resistance vessels, with flow reduced up to 50 per cent together with a loss of autoregulation. The precise cause of vasospasm is unknown, although it has been intensively investigated. In general, the more severe the bleed the greater the likelihood of subsequent vasospasm.

Box 4.4. Target values for triple H therapy

Haematocrit	30 per cent
CVP	10–12 mmHg
PA wedge pressure	15–18 mmHg
Systolic arterial pressure	160–200 mmHg
	120–150 mmHg (if aneurysm not clipped)

Prevention
Prevention of vasospasm is based on two factors: first, the correction of hypovolaemia with i.v. 0.9 per cent sodium chloride solution (see above); and secondly, the administration of the Ca^{2+} channel-blocking drug nimodipine (e.g. 60 mg orally 4-hourly). Nimodipine causes less systemic hypotension than other Ca^{2+} channel blockers, results in no difference in fluid and anaesthetic requirements, but obtunds autoregulation.

Treatment
Treatment of the vasospasm is based on the 'triple H' therapy of:

- Hypervolaemia
- Haemodilution
- Hypertension.

Hypertension may be difficult to attain if the aneurysm is not clipped. Measurement of the CVP is mandatory for triple H therapy, and often a pulmonary artery flotation catheter is required. It is usual to infuse colloid and crystalloid to expand the intravascular volume, and typical target values are shown in Box 4.4.

If volume expansion alone is insufficient to achieve the target figures, a vasopressor such as dopamine or noradrenaline is infused. Induced hypertension is necessary because autoregulation is lost. The complications of triple H therapy can be life threatening, and include myocardial ischaemia, pulmonary oedema and rebleeding of an unclipped aneurysm.

Anaesthetic considerations
In most units a SAH is operated on within 2–3 days of bleeding. This reflects the time to transfer from a referring hospital and the time taken to arrange angiography.

The primary consideration in anaesthesia for aneurysm clipping is control of the arterial pressure. Sudden increases in blood pressure must be prevented, as they increase the likelihood of rupture of the aneurysm. In addition, any major fall in blood pressure is deleterious as it compromises CBF.

Preoperative management

Careful preparation of patients is essential before aneurysm clipping. The key features are as follows:

- Use i.v. fluids to prevent hypovolaemia
- Control arterial pressure – aim for systolic pressure of 120–150 mmHg
- Give nimodipine
- Check ECG for arrhythmias and signs of ischaemia (? beta blockers)
- Clinically grade SAH
- Check CT scan
- Ask if there is evidence of vasospasm on angiography, or look for clinical signs
- Check for pulmonary oedema.

Maintenance of anaesthesia

- Use nitrous oxide/oxygen/isoflurane
- Ventilate the lungs to achieve a $PaCO_2$ of 4 kPa.

Monitoring

- Direct measurement of arterial pressure is mandatory
- CVP
- Urinary catheter.

Control of cerebral contents:

- Lumbar drain to remove CSF, and/or mannitol (neither to be used until skull flap is lifted).

Control of arterial pressure:

- i.v. fluids for hypotension
- Vasoactive drugs for hypertension (e.g. labetalol).

Postoperative care

Elective ventilation is occasionally necessary with difficult surgery. Maintain the systolic BP at 140–160 mmHg, and be aware of late onset vasospasm (see above).

Cerebral arteriovenous malformations

These often present as a SAH and attempts are usually made to embolize part of the malformation before surgery. At surgery the main complications are excessive bleeding, ischaemia in the area of brain around the malformation, and normal perfusion pressure breakthrough. This last term describes the oedema or haemorrhage that occurs in surrounding brain after surgical or embolic obliteration of the malformation, during which blood is shunted into local abnormally dilated vessels that previously surrounded the malformation.

5

Anaesthesia for tumour resection

Anaesthesia for supratentorial tumours, particularly for biopsy and debulking of malignant tumours, is usually undertaken with the basic neuroanaesthetic technique described in Chapter 3. However, two tumours merit additional discussion; pituitary tumours and meningiomas.

Pituitary tumours

Pituitary tumours usually present with visual field defects, but if the tumour extends above the pituitary fossa then the effects of a space-occupying lesion may be present, with impairment of hypothalamic function. Typically those tumours presenting with eye signs are non-secretory, whereas a secretory tumour usually presents with the effects of excessive hormone secretion while still very small in size. Surgery is increasingly conducted via a transphenoidal approach, as this provides the least risk of brain damage and haemorrhage. Occasionally a supratentorial approach is necessary. Anaesthetic management of a transphenoidal endonasal hypophysectomy is as follows.

Preoperative assessment
Assess carefully for:

- Acromegaly
- Diabetes mellitus
- Hypertension
- Diabetes insipidus
- Hypothyroidism
- Adrenal insufficiency.

There is often a complete endocrinological evaluation, but this may be out of date.

The airway must be assessed very carefully if the patient is acromegalic. Fibre-optic tracheal intubation may be indicated.

Ensure that steroid cover is started if indicated.

Induction of anaesthesia

- Direct measurement of arterial pressure is essential and CVP measurement advisory
- Insert urinary catheter
- Insert lumbar drain – injection of saline at the end of surgery enables the surgeon to ensure that tumour removal is complete
- Insert pharyngeal pack.
- Instil a vasoconstrictor such as cocaine (total dose 250 mg) into the nose to reduce bleeding. The surgeon also injects the submucosa with adrenaline solutions. This combination may cause hypertension and arrhythmias.

Maintenance of anaesthesia

- Carefully control the arterial pressure to aid the surgeon using the operating microscope
- There is always the risk of massive haemorrhage from the cavernous sinus or carotid artery.

Emergence from anaesthesia

- Remove the pharyngeal pack carefully
- Do not disturb the nasal packs placed by the surgeon
- Perform a thorough and careful pharyngeal toilet
- Extubate when very light.

Postoperative management

Standard postoperative care (see Chapter 10) plus:

- Check repeatedly for airway problems in acromegalics
- Continue steroids
- Look for CSF leak and nasal bleeding.

Diabetes insipidus occurs and may last for up to 10 days. The fluid input must be increased to match the loss, and vasopressin may be required.

Meningiomas

The main problem associated with the removal of these tumours is their extreme vascularity. Cerebral oedema is also common postoperatively. Blood loss during surgery can be diminished by preoperative embolization of massive tumours and the use of moderate hypotension during surgery. Rapid blood loss is particularly likely when the bone flap is raised and during removal of a bulky tumour. The anaesthetic technique for excision of a meningioma is the basic technique described in Chapter 3. However, direct measurement of the arterial pressure and CVP is mandatory, and sufficient large-bore venous cannulae must be inserted to cope with massive blood loss. A urinary catheter is also essential. Clotting problems may arise after surgery, either as a consequence of a large volume transfusion or because of the development of disseminated intravascular coagulation.

6

Anaesthesia for posterior fossa surgery

Most tumours in children arise in the posterior fossa. In adults, surgery in the posterior fossa is usually undertaken for tumours (such as an acoustic neuroma), aneurysms, arteriovenous abnormalities, and decompression of cranial nerves. The conduct of the anaesthetic is as described for a basic neuroanaesthetic technique in Chapter 3. There are, however, some additional problems that are more common in posterior fossa surgery (see Box 6.1).

Air embolism
Anaesthetists devoted much attention in the past to the problem of air embolism, and this probably reflected the common use of the sitting position of the patient for posterior fossa surgery. In many neurosurgical centres the sitting position is now used rarely, and the difficulties caused by air embolism have become trivial and infrequent.

The incidence is:

- 8 per cent – lateral position
- 10 per cent – supine position
- 25 per cent – sitting position.

The origin of the air is:

- The dural vessels
- The dural sinuses

Box 6.1. Problems in posterior fossa surgery

- Air embolism
- Damage to vital medullary centres
- Cranial nerve damage
- Positioning of the patient.

- The initial burr hole
- Vessels of the lesion.

Eighty per cent of air embolisms occur at the start of surgery, and 15 per cent at the end of surgery.

Physiological effects

The severity of the physiological effects is proportional to the volume of air and its rate of entry. Effects include:

- Pulmonary hypertension
- V/Q abnormality
- Cardiovascular collapse
- Arrhythmias
- Pulmonary oedema.

The obstruction to the right ventricular outflow tract produced by the air increases pressures in the right side of the heart and results in a decrease in arterial pressure. The consequent pulmonary V/Q mismatch is shown by an increase in $PaCO_2$ with a decrease in end-tidal PCO_2 and a decrease in PaO_2. If air passes to the left side of the heart, either through a patent foramen ovale or spillover through the lungs, then arterial air emboli can occur in the cardiac and cerebral circulations with disastrous consequences. If there is sufficient air in the right side of the heart, a 'mill-wheel' murmur may be heard with an oesophageal stethoscope. The relative sensitivity of the available monitors is listed in Box 6.2.

Box 6.2. Monitors for the detection of air embolism

More specific monitors of air embolism are:
- Doppler ultrasound over right heart
- End-tidal CO_2 measurement
- CVP or pulmonary artery (PA) catheter.

Less specific monitors of air embolism are:
- ECG
- Arterial pressure
- Oxygen saturation
- Oesophageal stethoscope.

Box 6.3. Recognition of air embolism

Early signs:

- Sound of air being aspirated, noted usually by surgeon!
- Change in doppler signal
- Decreased end-tidal CO_2
- Increased $PaCO_2$
- Decreased PaO_2
- Increased CVP or PA pressure.

Late signs:

- Decreased arterial pressure
- Arrhythmias
- Mill-wheel murmur.

Prevention

The decreasing prevalence of air embolism is due, in part, to the measures undertaken by the surgeon and anaesthetist.

Surgical measures include:

- Only using the sitting position when essential
- Sealing bone edges with wax
- Control of venous bleeding
- Irrigation of the surgical field.

Anaesthetic measures include:

- Avoiding the use of nitrous oxide
- Ensuring that the patient is well hydrated
- Using controlled ventilation.

It is important to note that if nitrous oxide is used as part of the anaesthetic technique then it will increase the volume of air by at least three-fold as the anaesthetic gas enters the air bubbles. Early diagnosis of air embolism allows prompt treatment. Cardiovascular changes occur late (see Box 6.3).

If cardiac arrest occurs, then a thoracotomy is necessary to aspirate the air from the right ventricle. Closed chest cardiac massage is rarely successful.

Treatment

Fortunately, most cases of air embolism are mild. If air embolism is detected, then further aspiration of air must be prevented. Treatment is undertaken as follows:

- Inform surgeon
- Start controlled ventilation if this is not already in use
- Increase the CVP
- Stop nitrous oxide, if necessary, and give 100 per cent O_2
- Try to aspirate air from the CVP or PA catheter (usually unsuccessful).

If air embolism is severe, or is only recognized late, additional procedures include placing the patient horizontal if anaesthetized in the sitting position, rapid i.v. infusion to raise the venous pressure, and treatment of cardiac arrhythmias if necessary.

Damage to vital medullary centres
Ischaemia of these centres is usually shown by changes in arterial pressure, heart rate and rhythm. Direct measurement of arterial pressure is essential for posterior fossa surgery. The cardiovascular disturbances usually resolve rapidly when surgical manipulation or retraction cease. Traction on the tenth nerve causes a bradycardia, and manipulation around the fifth nerve can lead to hypertension.

It was common to maintain spontaneous respiration for posterior fossa surgery in order to use respiratory changes as a warning of brainstem ischaemia. The advantages of controlled ventilation (see above) are now considered to be much greater than any possible benefit of using spontaneous respiration to monitor brainstem function.

Cranial nerve damage
The facial nerve is particularly at risk during the resection of an acoustic neuroma. It is usual to monitor facial nerve activity by direct intracranial stimulation of the nerve with electromyographic recording. The latter is converted to an audible signal, which enables the nerve to be identified and preserved during dissection of the tumour.

Positioning of the patient
Three positions may be used for posterior fossa surgery; the sitting position, prone position, and lateral recumbent (or 'park bench') position. The sitting position, which is used only occasionally, has the advantages of improved surgical access to midline tumours and decreased blood loss. However, disadvantages include:

- Cardiovascular instability
- Decreased cerebral perfusion with ischaemia
- Air embolism (see above)
- Airway obstruction (subglottic oedema and macroglossia)
- Pneumoencephalus
- Quadriplegia.

The lateral recumbent, or 'park bench', position is particularly appropriate for the resection of an acoustic neuroma, and is associated with a low incidence of air embolism.

Anaesthetic considerations

Preoperative care

- Patients are very sensitive to opiates, which must not be used
- Ensure adequate hydration if the sitting position is to be used
- The sitting position is contraindicated in: patent foramen ovale or ventriculo-atrial shunt; elderly and/or debilitated patients; cardiovascular instability; dehydration
- Preoperative contrast echocardiography may be used to screen for patent foramen ovale.

Induction and maintenance of anaesthesia

- Check position of the tracheal tube after positioning the patient
- Avoid using nitrous oxide
- Insert lumbar drain
- Use facial nerve monitoring for acoustic neuroma surgery
- Insert a urinary catheter
- Use methods for detection of air embolism (see above)
- Use slow staged positioning or 'G' suit to minimize hypotension in the sitting position.

Neuromuscular blocking drugs must be given by infusion and a peripheral nerve stimulator used to assess neuromuscular blockade. Facial nerve stimulation will not work if complete paralysis is present. At least two twitches must be seen on train-of-four stimulation, and all four should be present after tetanic stimulation.

Emergence from anaesthesia

It is imperative to check that protective laryngeal and pharyngeal reflexes are present on extubation.

Postoperative considerations

Damage to the ninth, tenth and eleventh cranial nerves can cause problems with swallowing, respiratory obstruction and depressed laryngeal reflexes. A period of tracheal intubation and ventilation may be necessary. Neurosurgical problems include bleeding, cerebral oedema, CSF leak and hydrocephalus.

7

Anaesthesia for spinal surgery

Surgery is indicated to relieve pressure on the spinal cord or nerve roots. Typical pathologies include disc lesions, spinal canal stenosis, tumours, and occasionally haematomas and abscesses. Anaesthesia for these problems is usually relatively simple in the thoracic and lumbar region, but more challenging in the cervical area. However, thoracic pathology may necessitate an anterior approach through a thoracotomy. Occasionally anaesthesia is needed for patients with acute spinal cord injury, and careful management of the patient is essential to avoid exacerbating cord ischaemia.

Spinal cord blood flow is controlled in a similar way to CBF, and the autoregulation curves for brain and spinal cord flow are very similar.

Basic anaesthetic technique

The basic anaesthetic technique for surgery in the thoracic and lumbar regions is as follows.

Preoperative considerations
- Note the intake of non-steroidal anti-inflammatory drugs (NSAIDs)
- Opioids may be needed for analgesia.

Induction of anaesthesia
- Use standard induction agent, opioid, non-depolarizing neuromuscular blocking drug technique
- Careful positioning of the patient on the operating table will help to keep the venous pressure low at the site of surgery.

Maintenance of anaesthesia
- Use volatile supplementation
- Use i.v. opioid (e.g. fentanyl)
- Maintain paralysis to prevent any movement.

Postoperative care

There is a wide variation in analgesia requirements.

Although many orthopaedic surgeons monitor spinal cord function with somatosensory and motor evolved responses during surgery on the spine, most neurosurgeons do not utilize physiological monitoring. Extensive experience indicates that this optimistic approach is justifiable.

Anaesthesia for cervical spine surgery

Anaesthesia for cervical spine surgery is similar to that described above, but there may be instability of the spine so that the patient must be anaesthetized wearing a cervical collar, or movement of the spine may be so restricted that fibre-optic intubation is indicated. Occasionally a transoral approach is necessary for cervical spine surgery, particularly for atlanto-axial instability. The airway is usually secured with a nasotracheal tube, although sometimes a tracheostomy is required. Transoral surgery can cause severe anaesthetic problems, and these include:

• Tracheal displacement with airway obstruction
• Puncture of the cuff on the tracheal tube
• Carotid artery compression
• Vocal cord paralysis.

Acute cord compression

Trauma to the cord disrupts autoregulation of spinal cord blood flow. The immediate systemic effects of cord ischaemia are:

• Brief hypertension followed by hypotension
• Bradycardia, with or without arrhythmias
• Decreased myocardial contractility with increased pulmonary artery wedge pressure
• Hypoxaemia.

These effects are similar to those found after a sudden marked increase in ICP.

Immediate management of patients with acute spinal cord injury

This may be summarized as follows:

• Identify the site of the injury, immobilize and transport the patient

- Respiration – check airway, give oxygen, prevent hypercarbia, intubate and ventilate lungs if necessary
- Circulation – maintain arterial pressure
- Assess associated injuries
- Attempt to preserve spinal cord function

Phases of spinal cord injury

There are several phases of spinal cord injury, and those most relevant to anaesthesia after acute cord injury are shown in Box 7.1.

The main clinical problems of the acute phase of cord injury are respiratory, cardiovascular and autonomic hyperreflexia.

Respiratory

An adequate airway with good oxygenation is essential to decrease the likelihood of hypoxia of the cord.

Cardiovascular

The initial hypertensive response to injury is not usually seen in clinical practice because it is short-lived. The common presentation is hypotension, bradycardia and supraventricular tachycardias.

Box 7.1 Phases of spinal cord injury

Acute (1–2 days after injury):
- Spinal shock
- Lower arterial pressure, Bradycardia
- Hypovolaemia
- Cord injury still evolving
- Nature and severity of other injuries not known
- Risk from full stomach.

Subacute (2 days to 1–12 weeks after injury):
- Spinal shock
- Risk of hyperkalaemia after suxamethonium
- Risk of hypercalcaemia.

Intermediate (1–12 weeks):
- Spinal shock resolved
- Hyperreflexia and possible spasm
- Autonomic hyperreflexia
- Severe risk of hyperkalaemia after suxamethonium
- Risk of hypercalcaemia.

Only lesions above T4 result in serious problems. This is thought to occur because cervical and high thoracic damage disrupts the sympathetic innervation of the heart, leaving vagal tone to predominate.

Autonomic hyperreflexia
After days, or sometimes weeks, reflexes below the level of the injury return. However, they are not localized and there is often a massive response to a mild stimulus. Signs include:

- Paroxysmal hypertension
- Arrhythmias
- Sweating
- Vasodilation above and vasoconstriction below the level of injury
- Anserina ('goose flesh').

Treatment of acute cord injury
Pharmacological treatment: Methylprednisolone 30 mg/kg i.v. is administered as soon as possible after the injury. In some centres large doses of dexamethasone are used. Mannitol or a loop diuretic is sometimes given, but there is no evidence to indicate their effectiveness.

Physical treatment: Cooling has been shown to be beneficial in animal models.

Surgical treatment: Surgery may be necessary to reduce and stabilize fracture/dislocations of the vertebrae.

Practical anaesthetic management
Anaesthesia is sometimes needed for cervical spine stabilization in patients with acute cord injury. It is essential that the patient is adequately resuscitated and the neck immobilized before anaesthesia is started.

The main controversy surrounds the method used to secure tracheal intubation. It must be assumed that the patient with a cord injury has a full stomach for many hours after the trauma. The choice is to use either an awake fibre-optic technique or a conventional rapid sequence induction with suxamethonium. The former is the method of choice if the anaesthetist is experienced with this technique; otherwise a rapid sequence induction with manual inline axial traction is safe and in the authors' unit has never been associated with inducing a neurological deficit. Suxamethonium is safe for 48–72 hours after spinal cord injury and should be used, as it provides the best conditions for intubation.

Anaesthesia should be continued in the conventional way with meticulous attention to the maintenance of cardiovascular stability and good oxygenation to minimize cord ischaemia. Full neuromuscular blockade provides the best and safest operating conditions. Postoperative care must be undertaken in ICU.

8

Anaesthesia for neuroimaging

Few radiological procedures are painful, and improvements in imaging techniques and equipment mean that patients rarely require anaesthesia. However, there is an increasing demand for an anaesthetic presence in the neuroradiology suite. This may be to provide sedation or general anaesthesia, to supervise ventilated intensive care patients during their investigations, or to help treat anaphylactic reactions to contrast media or the neurological complications of investigations. In addition, the continued development of interventional radiology makes new demands on the anaesthetist.

Anaesthesia in the radiology suite

For the anaesthetist the radiology department is an alien environment and presents potential problems with providing general anaesthesia. These difficulties are both physical and anaesthetic (see Box 8.1), and should be remembered whether anaesthesia is

---

Box 8.1. Potential problems for the anaesthetist in the radiology department

Physical considerations:

- Isolated site
- Limited space
- Poor lighting
- Cold
- Radiation hazards.

Anaesthetic considerations:

- Patient selection – often at the extremes of age or very sick
- Normal monitoring standards and full resuscitation equipment must be available
- Skilled assistance must be available
- Procedures are often long
- Patient movement
- Contrast media reactions.

---

required in the angiography suite, for computerized tomography (CT) or for magnetic resonance imaging (MRI).

Physical considerations

- The radiology suite is an isolated site often some distance from theatres, and provision for recovery and transportation must be made.
- Space is limited – there is often little room due to bulky equipment, and access to the patient may be restricted.
- Lighting is often dimmed and the room kept cool to prevent equipment overheating.
- Radiation hazards – adequate protective clothing (0.35 mm lead-equivalent aprons) must be worn, and the anaesthetist should always keep as far as possible from the radiation source during imaging. Radiation scatter decreases with increasing distance from the source (the inverse square law).

Anaesthetic considerations

- Patients' clinical status will depend on the underlying pathology and any pre-existing disease processes. They may be completely well or cerebrally obtunded and haemodynamically unstable, as following a subarachnoid haemorrhage or major head injury.
- Normal monitoring standards should be applied and anaesthetic equipment must be regularly serviced and maintained. Full resuscitation equipment must be available.
- Radiology personnel are rarely trained to provide anaesthetic help, and an appropriately skilled assistant must be available.
- Patient movement – there is frequent movement of the imaging table and of the X-ray tube. All connections to the patient must be secured and have sufficient slack to allow for this movement.
- Contrast media – reactions are relatively common, with reported incidences of between 2 and 5 per cent. Symptoms range from mild skin rashes, nausea and urticaria to anaphyl-actoid shock with hypotension, wheezing and cardiovascular collapse. Reactions are more common in atopic individuals, those with other allergies, or patients with cardiac disease. Pretreatment with steroids and antihistamines, at least 18 hours beforehand, has been shown to reduce the incidence in these patients. As with all anaphylaxis, the mainstay of treatment is epinephrine. All contrast media, except that used for MRI, contain iodine. The newer non-ionic, lower osmolality media have a lower incidence of

adverse reactions, but their increased cost precludes their routine use.

Interventional neuroradiology

There has been enormous progress in the field of interventional radiology over the last decade, and the dramatic increase in activity led the National Confidential Enquiry into Perioperative Deaths (NCEPOD) 2000 to devote a special report to the morbidity and mortality associated with it. The most common procedure performed is the therapeutic embolization of cerebral aneurysms. Therapeutic embolization is also used for embolization of cerebral or spinal arteriovenous malformations and vascular lesions, and may be used to reduce vascularity of tumours before surgery. Other indications include sclerotherapy of venous angiomas, intra-arterial chemotherapy of head and neck tumours, angioplasty, thrombolysis, and the pharmacotherapy of vasospasm.

The aim is to treat central nervous system pathology by endovascular placement of drugs or embolic material. A large sheath (7.5 Fr gauge) is placed (usually) in the femoral artery, through which a microcatheter is introduced and advanced under fluoroscopic guidance into the area to be treated. When the tip of the microcatheter is correctly placed, embolizing coils/glue, balloons, cytotoxic agents, thrombolytics or sclerotic drugs can be placed where needed. The Guglielmi detachable platinum microcoil (GDC) is soldered at the end of an insulated stainless steel guide wire. When it is correctly positioned it is detached by passing a current through it.

Preoperative assessment

The patient should have the same preoperative assessment as for neurosurgery. The prognosis depends on the neurological grading based on the GCS rather than the ASA grading. Points of particular relevance are previous problems with angiography, reactions to contrast material, coagulation disorders, and any conditions that might make lying still for several hours very difficult – e.g. a confused patient, airway problems, or neck, back or joint disorders. In patients with intracranial vascular pathology the potential complications are understandably very frightening, and premedication may minimize hypertension secondary to apprehension. Some patients, for example those with large arteriovenous malformations (AVM), will need multiple procedures, and patient acceptability is of great importance. Some centres use nimodipine prophylaxis for prevention of cerebral vasospasm.

Sedation

Local anaesthesia and sedation often provide good conditions and preserve the ability to assess the patient neurologically during the procedure. However, traction or distension of vessels can cause pain, and discomfort from prolonged periods of lying motionless can be a real problem. In addition, for very long procedures large amounts of sedation may be needed, with the risk of respiratory depression and carbon dioxide retention. In these cases, general anaesthesia should be considered.

The aims are to alleviate anxiety and patient discomfort, and to provide analgesia. Intermittent neurological assessment is often needed, and so sedation should be easily reversible. Neurolept anaesthesia (fentanyl and droperidol) or incremental doses of midazolam (1 mg boluses) and fentanyl (25 μg boluses) have been used successfully. However, neither are ideal for long cases. Propofol infusions provide good conditions and easily titratable sedation. Supplemental oxygen is essential for all patients, and airway obstruction must be avoided.

Immediate intervention may be required if a disaster (such as intracranial haemorrhage) occurs, and the anaesthetist must be prepared for this. Good communication between the neuroradiologist and anaesthetist is vital.

General anaesthesia

General anaesthesia is required for children, for uncooperative patients and for certain procedures, such as aneurysm ablation, when the patient needs to be absolutely motionless. Anaesthetic considerations and choice of drugs follow the general principles of neuroanaesthesia. Neuroradiological procedures are less painful and are usually without significant blood loss. However, it is just as important to ensure smooth anaesthesia and the avoidance of cerebral vasodilating drugs. When patients undergo craniotomy the brain is decompressed, so they are protected to a certain extent from rises in intracranial pressure (ICP). This does not happen in the angiography suite.

Drugs

Intravenous anaesthesia with propofol is a reasonable choice, as its rapid recovery allows immediate neurological assessment. Fentanyl or remifentanil provide analgesia, and an infusion of vecuronium or atracurium is used for muscle relaxation. Because of its effects on cerebral haemodynamics and the presence of air bubbles in the arterial circulation, nitrous oxide is often avoided.

Ventilation
Controlled ventilation to moderate hypocapnia has been reported to have a beneficial effect on the quality of films in cerebral angiography. The resultant slowing of the cerebral circulation allows more images to be taken during the arterial phase of the angiogram. In addition, vasoconstriction allows the contrast medium to fill the arterial lumen and provides better definition.

Monitoring
This should include direct arterial pressure, ECG and pulse oximetry (it has been suggested that the instrument for measuring this should be placed on the toe of the leg in which the femoral sheath is inserted to give an early indication of femoral artery obstruction or embolization). Cardiovascular instability can occur during the procedure. Periods of apnoea or hypercapnia may be requested, and end-tidal carbon dioxide monitoring and an apnoea alarm are mandatory. A temperature probe should be used and measures taken to maintain normothermia. At least one large-bore intravenous cannula should be sited with a long extension and three-way tap distant from the patient, to maximize distance between the anaesthetist and the fluoroscopy unit. A urinary catheter is advisable, as large volumes of flush solution are used.

Anticoagulation
Heparin is usually given during the procedure to prevent thromboembolic complications. A baseline measurement of the activated clotting time (ACT) is made after femoral artery cannulation, and the aim is to provide an ACT of at least twice the baseline. Following an uncomplicated procedure protamine may be given to reverse anticoagulation, but often anticoagulation is continued to prevent thrombosis distal to the treated area.

Blood pressure control
Induced hypotension/hypertension may be required. This might be to test the safety of carotid occlusion or to keep glue in place within an AVM, and may be for relatively short periods of time but several episodes may be necessary. Agents of choice should have minimal

effects on the cerebral vasculature. Labetalol has been used successfully, as has esmolol.

Postoperative care
At the end of the procedure the catheter is removed and pressure applied to the groin to prevent haematoma formation; the patient may then be extubated. On emergence, appropriate measures must be taken to avoid coughing, hypertension etc. For all intracranial, procedures the patient is usually monitored on the neurosurgical intensive care unit for the next 24 hours.

Complications
The complication rate varies with the procedure performed, but has been reported to be as high as 20 per cent. Complications include:

- Intracranial haemorrhage (2–3 per cent of cases). This may occur as a result of leakage of an acute aneurysm, or vessel rupture in an AVM or normal vessel. It results in marked haemodynamic instability, typically bradycardia and hypertension. Treatment is by control of the blood pressure and reversal of anticoagulation. If the haemorrhage is slight, coil placement may be continued. If it is severe, management is for spontaneous subarachnoid haemorrhage following transfer to the intensive care unit.
- Cerebral ischaemia. This may occur during catheter manipulation or secondary to misplaced injectate (e.g. coil or glue).
- Thromboembolic complications.
- Groin haematoma.

Computed tomography
Although magnetic resonance imaging (MRI) has largely superseded computerized tomography (CT) scanning, it is still the main radiographic tool for examination of structures within the body cavities and in the emergency situation. CT is still recommended as the primary diagnostic imaging method in the patient with an acute head injury or multiple trauma. General anaesthesia guarantees a motionless patient with a secure airway, and may be necessary in children and in unconscious or uncooperative patients.

Sedation
Small babies will sleep through even long procedures if they are well wrapped up and the study is performed after feeding. However, up

to 80 per cent of infants are sedated for CT scanning. Sedation is usually carried out by a radiologist, and many different regimens are available. Chloral hydrate is still commonly used, and midazolam is also popular. However, if sedation fails the child often has to return for general anaesthesia. Excessive sedation carries the risk of hypoxia as a result of airway compromise or respiratory depression. The provision of an anaesthetist solely for supervision of sedation is unfeasible. Guidelines have been issued by a joint working party of the Royal College of Anaesthetists and the Royal College of Radiologists. Recommendations include secure venous access, and monitoring with pulse oximetry, ECG and blood pressure. Oxygen and resuscitation equipment should be available, and staff involved should be trained in cardiopulmonary resuscitation.

General anaesthesia
If general anaesthesia is indicated because of multiple trauma, these patients must be stabilized before being moved to the X-ray department. Otherwise, the anaesthetic technique should be that appropriate for the patient.

Magnetic resonance imaging
Magnetic resonance imaging is now clearly established as the imaging technique of choice in the investigation of the central nervous system, and as its applications continue to expand so the need for sedation and anaesthesia is also increasing. The presence of high-strength magnetic fields and radiofrequency waves makes this a particularly challenging environment for the anaesthetist to work in, and has major implications regarding patient safety. Anaesthetists must have a basic understanding of the principles of MRI.

MRI-sensitive nuclei, such as hydrogen, possess a property known as spin. When these nuclei are placed in an extrinsic magnetic field, they align themselves with that magnetic field. They continue to spin, but their axis of rotation moves around the axis of the magnetic field. If they are then subjected to a second, transient magnetic field oscillating at their resonant frequencies (usually in the radiofrequency range) and orientated at right angles to the first magnetic field, they are deflected. When the radiofrequency pulse is removed, the nuclei rotate back into alignment with the static magnetic field and energy is released. This energy is converted to produce a magnetic resonance image. Clinical MRI pictures are produced by mapping the signal from hydrogen nuclei in tissue water.

Technical considerations

Magnetic field

Magnetic field strength is measured in tesla (T) or gauss (G), where 1 tesla is equal to 10 000 gauss. MRI units in clinical practice usually operate at between 0.5–2.0 T, but some newer systems are as high as 4 T. Anaesthetists need to be aware of the extent of the magnetic field they are working in. The greater the magnetic field, the better the resolution of the images but the greater the associated technical problems. The magnetic field is maximal at the magnet bore, but extends beyond, gradually decreasing in strength (fringe field). Useful measures in practice are the 50 G and 5 G lines. At the 5 G line electrical equipment may malfunction, pacemakers may dysfunction and computer disks may be erased. The magnet should be considered to be permanently on.

Ferromagnetic attraction

The attractive force on ferromagnetic objects becomes significant at field strengths of about 50 G. Oxygen cylinders and scissors have the potential to become dangerous missiles, and ferromagnetic objects must be positioned outside the 50 G line or firmly secured to the walls or floor. Persons entering the MRI suite must actively check for and remove such objects. All units operate patient exclusion criteria and have comprehensive checklists.

The MRI compatibility and safety of artificial implants is a particular problem. Many are non-ferromagnetic, and others will pose little threat if they are very small or firmly fixed (e.g. joint prostheses). However, movement of others (e.g. cerebral aneurysm clips or intraocular foreign bodies) could be disastrous. Useful information about the properties of implants can be obtained from reviews or Internet websites (see Box 8.2). Patients should never be taken for MRI scanning if there is any doubt about their safety. Pacemakers, automatic defibrillators, cochlear implants and implanted drug infusion devices will malfunction at much lower field strengths, and should not be taken into the MRI suite.

Biological effects of MRI

MRI appears to be safe. There is no ionizing radiation and no protective clothing need be worn. However, it has only been in

> **Box 8.2. Internet websites providing information on MRI compatibility**
>
> - UK Medical Devices Agency – http://www. medical-devices.gov.uk/
> - Magnetic resonance safety site –
>   http://kanal-arad.upmc.edu/mrsafety.html
> - Food and Drug Administration Center for Devices and Radiological Health – http://www.fda.gov/default.htm

use for a relatively short time, and caution must still be advised. Patients are exposed to three different types of radiation: the static magnetic field, a gradient magnetic field and radiofrequency magnetic field. Evidence from human studies suggests that static magnetic fields up to 2.5 T have no side effects. The gradient magnetic field is rapidly switching, and the electrophysiological effects can be significant at greater strengths. Radiofrequency electromagnetic fields induce currents in tissues, which can have significant heating effects. Concerns have been raised over adverse effects on the eye or testes, but evidence to date does not support these fears. Data regarding teratogenic effects are contradictory, but most units limit occupational exposure during pregnancy. There are few data on the safety of high-field (4–5 T) magnets.

Monitors

Reliable monitoring is as mandatory in the MRI suite as in the operating theatre, especially as access to the patient and visibility are limited. However, some modification of equipment may be necessary. The static magnetic field means that monitoring equipment must be kept away from the magnet. Both the gradient and the radiofrequency magnetic fields can induce currents and heat production in monitoring leads. These can not only result in device malfunction, but may also produce burns. Leads of monitoring equipment can act as aerials, which cause distortion of images. Specifically designed, compatible monitoring equipment should be used when possible to minimize problems. All ferrous components should be removed from leads and probes, or plastic/disposable ones used. All leads should be kept short and care taken to ensure that they do not form loops (e.g. by twisting or braiding). Fibre-optic cables should be used where possible. Various publications are available that list compatible equipment, and it should be noted that manufacturers classify their equipment as MR-safe (no harm to patients) or MR-compatible (safe and no mutual effect on the scanning process). The unavailability of specific equipment must not justify unsafe practice.

Noise

The gradient magnetic fields produce a loud thumping noise, and this means that MRI scanners are very noisy. Temporary hearing loss has been reported. To reduce noise levels, patients are fitted with MR-compatible earplugs.

Time

Despite technical advances, scans still take considerable time. A single image can take 20 minutes to obtain, and the whole process may last for over an hour. This means that general anaesthesia may be necessary for children and confused or uncooperative individuals.

Anaesthetic considerations

Many MRI suites were constructed without general anaesthesia in mind, and anaesthesia in a MRI unit should not be undertaken lightly. Lying motionless for long periods within the magnet bore makes many patients feel claustrophobic. This, in combination with the noise, means that up to 5 per cent of scans have to be aborted. Reassurance, counselling and, possibly, light sedation are usually sufficient in adults.

As with CT scans, small babies will sleep if they are warm and recently fed. More than 80 per cent of infants are sedated. Techniques and requirements follow the same rules as for CT scanning, but remembering the use of MR-compatible monitoring equipment. Care must be taken to avoid respiratory depression, especially in neurosurgical patients. Airway management is often easier under general anaesthesia than under deep sedation.

For failed sedation and uncooperative adults, general anaesthesia is necessary. Unconscious patients will need airway protection and controlled ventilation. Critically ill patients present a particular challenge in the MRI suite.

Considerations for anaesthesia for MRI are summarized in Box 8.3.

Box 8.3. Considerations for anaesthesia for MRI

Technical considerations:
- Magnetic field
- Ferromagnetic attraction
- Biological effects
- Noise.

Anaesthetic considerations:
- MRI-compatible equipment
- Time
- Patient selection.

Anaesthetic technique

The anaesthetic machine can be sited within the magnetic field, allowing the anaesthetist to stay close to the patient. An MRI-compatible machine and ventilator are necessary, or a firmly secured wall bar. Alternatively, the machine can be positioned at the edge of the magnetic field. Extra long lengths of breathing system and monitoring leads are required, with an increased risk of disconnection. Airway management depends on the individual patient. The laryngeal mask is widely used, and is a useful alternative to tracheal intubation. Reinforced laryngeal masks are ferromagnetic and produce distortion of the image, but there is a new version with a plastic spiral specifically for MRI. For intubation, preformed tracheal tubes such as the RAE tube are ideal, as there is little space when the head coils are in place. For maintenance, both volatile agents and intravenous anaesthesia have been used successfully. The patient may breathe spontaneously or be ventilated. Breathing systems should be lightweight, have no metal components, and have a low expiratory resistance. Infusion pumps may malfunction at 30 G, need long extension sets and must be mounted on non-ferromagnetic poles. Compatible trolleys are used. A suitable recovery area, appropriately equipped and staffed, should be available.

9

Monitoring of the central nervous system

Monitoring of CNS aims to detect changes in cerebral haemodynamics and oxygenation, and neuronal function. Advances in technology have enabled the development of many new monitors, some of which are already in clinical use. Despite these developments, cerebral function assessed by clinical examination and coupled with a detailed history still represents the gold standard. However in the perioperative period and on the intensive care unit clinical assessment is notoriously difficult and alternative methods are required.

Clinical assessment
The Glasgow Coma Scale
The Glasgow Coma Scale (GCS) provides a standardized and internationally accepted means of quantifying central nervous system (CNS) depression (Box 9.1). It is based on the patient's best response in terms of eye opening, motor response and verbal response. A patient scoring 8 or less is, by definition, in a coma.

Pupil size and reaction
Changes in pupil size and reaction provide additional information – for example, a fixed dilated pupil indicates compression of the third cranial nerve.

Cerebral perfusion and haemodynamics
Cerebral blood flow monitors can provide information on global and regional blood flow. Global information may be obtained by transcranial doppler ultrasonography, jugular bulb oxygen saturation and near infrared spectroscopy. Regional cerebral perfusion monitoring uses brain tissue oxygen monitoring and cerebral microdialysis.

Box 9.1. The Glasgow Coma Scale (GCS)

Eye opening	*(E score)*
Spontaneous	E = 4
To speech (not necessarily a request for eye opening)	E = 3
To pain (stimulus applied to face)	E = 2
None	E = 1
Best motor response	*(M score)*
Obeys commands	M = 6
Localizes (purposeful movement towards stimulus)	M = 5
Normal flexion (withdraws from stimulus)	M = 4
Abnormal flexion (decorticate posture)	M = 3
Extension (decerebrate posture)	M = 2
No movement	M = 1
Verbal response	*(V score)*
Orientated	V = 5
Confused	V = 4
Inappropriate words	V = 3
Incomprehensible sounds	V = 2
None	V = 1

Cerebral perfusion

The cerebral perfusion pressure (CPP) is defined as the difference between mean arterial pressure (MAP) and intracranial pressure (ICP):

$$CPP = MAP - ICP$$

A decrease in MAP or an elevation in ICP will decrease the effective perfusion pressure. In adults with head injury, treatment based on optimizing CPP has been shown to improve outcome and maintenance of a CPP >70 mmHg is recommended.

ICP monitoring

In addition to allowing calculation of CPP, ICP monitoring indicates changes in intracranial volume and can be used to guide treatments. ICP can be measured in a number of sites – epidural or subdural (subarachnoid, intraventricular or parenchymal). Each of these has recognized risks and benefits. An intraventricular catheter is the gold standard in terms of accuracy, and has the added advantage that it can be used for CSF drainage. However, its placement requires more skill and is associated with a higher incidence of infection and a greater potential for brain injury during placement. Subdural bolts, subdural catheters and intraparenchymal sensors can also be used. The catheters used may be a simple, fluid-filled transduced system, or fibre-optic devices.

Transcranial doppler ultrasonography
Transcranial doppler ultrasonography (TCD) provides inexpensive, continuous and non-invasive information on cerebral dynamics. TCD measures the velocity of the red blood cells flowing through the basal cerebral vessels. Using a range-gated, direction-sensitive ultrasound probe, the cerebral artery is insonated by a low frequency (2 MHz) pulsed wave through one of the three acoustic windows, the transtemporal, transorbital and transforminal. Transtemporal insonation allows examination of the middle (MCA), anterior (ACA) and posterior (PCA) arteries. The middle cerebral artery is the easiest to detect and carries about 75 per cent of the ipsilateral blood flow, making it representative of hemispheric blood flow.

The waveform obtained shows peak, diastolic and mean flow velocities. The TCD measures velocity, not flow. However, as the diameter of the basal cerebral vessels is unaffected by changes in blood pressure or $PaCO_2$, changes in flow velocity correlate closely with changes in flow. TCD is therefore used to monitor cerebral blood flow on the ITU and in anaesthetized patients. Anaesthetic agents may decrease CBF and consequently reduce TCD velocities. Marked changes are seen in patients with intracranial hypertension and during procedures such as carotid endarterectomy or balloon occlusion.

Dividing the difference between the systolic and diastolic velocities by the mean velocity derives the pulsatility index (PI). This has been shown to correlate better with cerebral perfusion pressure than ICP. Transcranial doppler ultrasonography not only monitors cerebral blood flow and cerebral perfusion; it is also useful in the diagnosis of vasospasm and to test cerebral autoregulation and vasoreactivity. It has been used as well to detect cerebral emboli during cardiac and neurovascular surgery.

Several technical difficulties exist. It is essential to keep the insonation depth and angle constant during the examination period, and maintenance of the probe position during surgery and in the ITU can be very difficult.

Cerebral oxygenation

Jugular bulb venous oximetry

Cerebral venous oxygenation (SJO_2) provides a global measure of the balance between cerebral blood flow (CBF) and oxygen consumption ($CMRO_2$). Venous blood from the brain drains into the cerebral sinuses. The final common pathway for the majority of the blood is through the right and left sigmoid sinuses and finally into the jugular bulbs. Under normal circumstances $CMRO_2$ matches the CBF, and the ratio between the two variables can be described by the arterial-jugular venous oxygen content difference ($AVDO_2$) according to the Fick principle:

$$AVDO_2 = CMRO_2/CBF$$

Assuming the amount of dissolved haemoglobin is negligible, total haemoglobin concentration (tHb) and the Hb dissociation constant and arterial oxygen saturation (SaO_2) remain unchanged over time, then the ratio of CBF to $CMRO_2$ is proportional to SJO_2.

Jugular bulb catheters are inserted by retrograde cannulation of the internal jugular vein. The catheter is inserted through the introducer and advanced until the tip is positioned at the base of the skull. The position of the catheter must be confirmed by X-ray (lateral cervical spine or antero-posterior chest including the neck). The end of the catheter should lie at the level of and just medial to the mastoid bone at the level of C1/C2. Contraindications and complication rates are similar to those for routine internal jugular access. To accurately reflect global and hemispheric blood flow, the dominant jugular bulb must be cannulated. Selecting the optimal side can be difficult. Usually flow is greater to the right jugular bulb, but this can be altered in patients with intracranial pathology. The dominant side of venous flow can be identified by the greater increase in ICP during unilateral jugular compression.

Cerebral venous oxygenation can be measured continuously using fibre-optic oximetric catheters or by intermittent blood sampling. Normal SJO_2 in healthy subjects ranges from 55 to 75 per cent. A decrease in SJO_2 indicates cerebral hypoperfusion, with oxygen demand exceeding supply. At SJO_2 values <40 per cent, increases in cerebral venous lactate concentrations indicate global cerebral ischaemia. Conversely, an increase in SJO_2 implies relative hyperaemia. Changes in haemoglobin, arterial blood gases, body temperature, ICP and administration of drugs will alter the readings. A number of technical factors also affect SJO_2; the optimal site of catheter placement is still unknown, and the catheter position affects the readings. The rate of blood withdrawal will also alter SJO_2. Faster withdrawal increases extracranial contamination and overestimates SJO_2 by 8–17 per cent – the optimal rate is 2 ml/min. The new modified fibre-optic catheters claim to have significant improvements and reduce the artefacts due to baseline drift and external light interference seen with some of the earlier catheters.

Despite these problems, SJO_2 monitoring has been used extensively in the management of head injury and during neurosurgical procedures. It is a useful tool in guiding therapy for intracranial hypertension following head injury. An optimal CPP can be defined as when an increase in arterial pressure produces no further increase in SJO_2. Hyperventilation is associated with a worse outcome after head injury and should be used with great care, but SJO_2 monitoring allows ventilation to be adjusted to provide optimal brain conditions.

Near infrared spectroscopy

Near infrared spectroscopy (NIRS) is a method for continuous non-invasive monitoring of cerebral saturation. It has been used for many years in neonatal intensive care. The technology is similar to that for pulse oximetry in that it follows a modified Beer–Lambert law. Light in the near infrared range (650–900 nm) can pass through skin, bone and other tissues relatively easily, but when passed through brain tissue it is partly scattered and partly absorbed. The amount of light absorbed is proportional to the concentrations of chromophores (oxyhaemoglobin, HbO_2; deoxyhaemoglobin, Hb; and cytochrome oxidase, CytOx). It is possible to measure brain oxygenation by quantifying the relative absorption of oxyhaemoglobin (HbO_2) and deoxyhaemoglobin (Hb) in the cerebral tissue. By using a modification of the Fick principle, changes in cerebral blood flow and cerebral blood volume can be detected. Normal values of HbO_2 are reported to be 60–80 per cent.

Only reflectance spectroscopy, when both emitting and receiving optodes are placed on the same side of the skull, is used in adults, as the large head and thick skull makes transmission spectroscopy (as used in neonates) impossible. The optodes are placed on one side of the forehead away from the midline (avoiding the cerebral sinuses and the temporalis muscle) and at an acute angle to each other, about 6 cm apart. A major concern is the inability of NIRS to distinguish between extracranial and intracranial changes in cerebral blood flow and oxygenation. The amount of extracranial contamination decreases with increasing interoptode distance. NIRS remains at present primarily a research tool, but clinical applications are emerging. NIRS has been used in patients with head injury or intracranial haemorrhage, and in patients undergoing carotid endarterectomy. Studies have demonstrated a close relationship between cerebral desaturation to values of less than 55 per cent and cerebral hypoperfusion or systemic hypoxia.

Brain tissue oxygen measurement
An alternative way to monitor cerebral oxygenation locally, in at risk areas of the brain, is by the use of probes to measure tissue PO_2. At the moment there are two types of sensor available commercially. The Licox sensor measures PO_2 and temperature continuously, via a miniaturized polargraphic Clark electrode and thermocouple incorporated within the tip of a microcatheter. The Neurotrend has additional microsensors to allow measurement of PCO_2 and pH. The sensors are placed in contact with cortical tissue during craniotomy or via a standard burr hole, but, despite being highly invasive, reports so far suggest that this monitoring is safe. Studies to date suggest that results are reliable and reproducible.

Cerebral microdialysis
Intracerebral microdialysis has been introduced recently, and at present is a research tool. Molecules such as glucose, lactate, glutamate, glycerol and urea can be extracted from the extracellular space. The principle is based on the passive transfer of substances across a dialysis membrane. Samples can be analysed within minutes of collection, providing instantaneous comparison with the clinical state of the patient. In patients with traumatic brain injury and subarachnoid haemorrhage, lactate and glutamate appear to be sensitive markers of impending ischaemia, whereas glycerol levels are associated with severe ischaemic deficits.

Monitoring of the central nervous system is summarized in Box 9.2.

Cerebral function monitoring
Brain electrical monitoring may be used to detect changes in neuronal function caused by ischaemia or neuronal damage following trauma. The electroencephalogram (EEG) and evoked potentials

---

Box 9.2. Monitoring of the central nervous system

- Intracranial pressure
- Cerebral perfusion – transcranial doppler (TCD)
- Cerebral oxygenation:
  - Jugular bulb venous oxygen saturation (SJO$_2$)
  - Near infra-red spectroscopy (NIRS)
  - Brain tissue oxygen
  - Microdialysis
- Neuronal function:
  - Electroencephalogram (EEG)
  - Cerebral function monitor (CFM)
  - Bispectral index (BIS)
  - Evoked potentials (EPs)

(EPs) respond rapidly to changes in cerebral physiology and provide a non-invasive means of assessing brain function.

The electroencephalogram

The electroencephalogram (EEG) represents brain electrical activity as recorded from the scalp, and is characterized by a complex pattern of voltage fluctuations. The scalp potentials recorded are thought to result from the summation of excitatory and inhibitory postsynaptic potentials from many pyramidal neurones. Functional abnormalities in subcortical brain structures induce characteristic changes in the surface EEG. The EEG is recorded using metal (usually silver) disc electrodes. These are arranged using an internationally recognized placement (the 10:20 electrode placement system). The signal is then amplified and filtered, which removes unwanted electrical activity. The EEG is displayed as a graph of voltage (amplitude) over time. It is characterized in terms of:

- Frequency of the background rhythm – δ (0.5–4 Hz), θ (4–8 Hz), α (8–13 Hz), β (>13 Hz)
- Amplitude (voltage) – most normal EEG activity is between 20 and 200 V
- Rhythms and patterns
- Symmetry or asymmetry
- Reactivity to sensory stimuli.

The normal EEG depends on the age and state of arousal, changing markedly during childhood. It produces a large amount of data that require specialist interpretation. Analysis is performed according to two fundamentally different techniques, based on analysis of frequency of the EEG signal over time, or amplitude over time. Power spectral analysis is one of the most commonly used frequency-based methods. One of the simplest methods of processing the EEG is the *cerebral function monitor* (CFM), which uses only one channel of data and filters and compresses it. The result is a single trace, which is dependent on both the amplitude and the frequency of the underlying EEG and is easily interpreted without extensive training.

The EEG changes in a predictable manner as the depth of anaesthesia is increased. Different agents produce characteristic effects on the EEG. Intraoperative EEG monitoring has gained widespread acceptance for carotid endarterectomy. On the ITU the EEG is useful in the diagnosis of certain conditions that have characteristic EEG changes, such as herpes simplex, measles encephalitis or Creutzfeld–Jakob. It is also used in the management of status epilepticus and in predicting outcome from coma.

The EEG as a depth of anaesthesia monitor has been the focus of attention for years, but the changes are usually biphasic and may also alter with different anaesthetic agents. A *BIS monitor* analyses the EEG by bispectral analysis (consisting of Fourier transformation and phase coupling studies) and then calculates the bispectral index (BIS) and many other variables. The bispectral index (BIS) provides a single figure that is a measure of CNS depression. In awake subjects the BIS is about 95, and the probability of awareness is extremely low when the BIS is less than 50. The monitor shows promise at predicting depth of anaesthesia.

Evoked potentials

Unlike the EEG, which represents spontaneous cortical activity, evoked potentials (EPs) are electrical potentials produced in response to stimulation of the nervous system by sensory, electrical, magnetic or cognitive means. Sensory evoked potentials (SEPs) are produced by stimulation of the sensory system. The responses arise from action potential propagation, or graded polysynaptic potentials, during the propagation of an electrical impulse from the periphery to the brain, and can be recorded from the scalp, as well as various sites along the anatomical pathway, using surface or subdermal electrodes. Auditory evoked potentials (AEPs) reflect the response of different areas of the brain to auditory stimuli, and visual evoked potentials (VEPs) are the cortical responses to visual stimulation. In contrast to the EEG, which represents the spontaneous activity of the cortex, these potentials are specific to the pathway and stimulus. The amplitudes of the electrical response are small (0.5–5 µV) when compared to the EEG, so computer averaging is used to extract the SEP signal from the background EEG noise. The number of stimuli required for the individual stimulus modality depends on the relative size of the response, ranging from 64 to 128 stimuli for SEP and VEP but more than 1000 for brainstem auditory evoked potentials (BAEPs). The EP waveforms are graded according to their amplitude and latency, and whether they are positive or negative (with respect to a reference zero).

Sensory evoked potentials
The largest experience is with monitoring of somatosensory evoked potentials (SSEP). A square-wave stimulus of 0.2–2 ms duration is delivered to a peripheral nerve (usually a mixed motor and sensory nerve such as the median or tibial nerve) and the intensity adjusted to produce a minimal muscle contraction (motor threshold). Intraoperative recordings of SSEPs have been used to assess functional integrity of sensory pathways during procedures in which they might be at risk, such as operations on the spine or spinal cord, and peripheral nerve surgery. An important limitation is the sensitivity of the cerebral responses to anaesthetic agents. For this reason recordings are often made from the spinal cord, as anaesthetic agents have less effect on spinal or subcortical SSEPs. SSEP monitoring has also been used during vascular surgery, carotid endarterectomy and interventional neuroradiology.

Brainstem auditory evoked responses
Brainstem auditory evoked responses are produced by a simple auditory stimulus, usually a click, and consist of a series of positive and negative waves, which represent the activation of the various relay structures from the cochlea to the brainstem and through to the cortex. BAEP monitoring may be used to assess brainstem function during posterior fossa surgery.

Visual evoked potentials
Visual evoked potentials monitor the function of the retina, optic chiasm and cortex, and radiation, and are recorded in response to flash stimuli applied using light emitting goggles or a checkerboard. They have very limited application in the operating theatre.

The different drugs used during anaesthesia and on the ITU can effect the monitoring of EPs; VEPs seem to be the most sensitive and BAEPs the least. Late potentials (cortical) are affected more than early waves (brainstem). Volatile anaesthetics affect spinal and subcortical waves less than cortical potentials.

Electrophysiological monitoring provides a method of assessing the functional integrity of vulnerable neural pathways in anaesthetized patients, and is considered mandatory in certain cases. However, the equipment is very expensive and interpretation is difficult.

10

Postoperative care

The monitoring and control of physiological variables is as important postoperatively as during surgery, and hence the majority of neurosurgical patients need to be managed in a high dependency or intensive care unit. Postoperative hypoxia or haemodynamic instability can have catastrophic effects on the brain, and even those patients with minimal neurological symptoms preoperatively may be difficult to assess postoperatively as a result of surgery or residual anaesthesia. Some patients, especially those in whom surgery has been complicated or prolonged, will need to be ventilated for several hours or overnight. Facilities for invasive cardiovascular monitoring, artificial ventilation, intracranial pressure measurement and central nervous system monitoring should be available. Close liaison between the anaesthetic team and the neurosurgeons is essential.

Monitoring

Clinical assessment by a trained neurosurgical nurse remains the most important monitor of neurological function. Assessment should include pupil size, limb strength, and the Glasgow Coma Score (GCS). Intracranial pressure monitoring is indicated in patients who have intracranial hypertension – especially if they are sedated, making clinical assessment difficult. Additional central nervous system monitoring is used if appropriate.

Direct arterial pressure monitoring is routine in all patients who have had intracranial procedures, and in ventilated patients. Central venous pressure monitoring is required in those who have cardiac disease, haemodynamic instability, or need vasoactive infusions. Pulmonary artery catheters may be useful in patients with cardiovascular disease or vasospasm.

Hourly urinary output and careful monitoring of fluid balance are very important. Neurosurgical patients are at risk of large fluid shifts and electrolyte imbalances as a result of the use of osmotic diuretics, or secondary to cerebral pathology. Full blood count, clotting screen and electrolytes should be measured regularly.

Sedation and analgesia

Postoperative pain is an important problem, and until recently was poorly managed for fear of masking neurological deterioration. Traditional teaching that morphine should be avoided in neurosurgical patients is now disputed. Regular paracetamol, non-steroidal anti-inflammatory drugs such as diclofenac (if there are no contraindications) and codeine phosphate are very useful, especially if given in adequate dosage. However, morphine is often necessary in the first 24 hours and can be used safely providing the patient is monitored. Nausea or vomiting should be treated aggressively.

Sedation may be needed to decrease anxiety, facilitate mechanical ventilation and attenuate responses to noxious stimuli. The ideal agent has no adverse effects on cerebral haemodynamics, but also allows rapid recovery to enable neurological assessment to be undertaken. Propofol is now widely used.

Fluid management

Traditionally neurosurgical patients have been fluid restricted to minimize the risk of cerebral oedema, despite the scant evidence to support this. However, there is some evidence from serum osmolalities in postoperative craniotomy patients given typical maintenance fluids (30–35 ml/kg per day) that these contain excess water and that moderate fluid restriction may prevent hypo-osmotically driven oedema. On the other hand, hypovolaemia or hypotension will lead to a reduction in cerebral blood flow, especially to 'at risk' areas of the brain. Therefore, fluid administration should aim to maintain normovolaemia and a normal serum osmolality.

Those patients who have had intracranial vascular surgery require a hyperdynamic circulation, as in the management of vasospasm. In this group of patients, 3 l daily, of which one is colloid, is usually sufficient.

The choice of fluids is still the subject of debate. The available data suggest that the type of fluid replacement will have no effect on cerebral oedema providing normal serum osmolality is maintained. Perioperative fluid replacement usually consists of 0.9 per cent sodium chloride solution.

Glucose-containing solutions are generally avoided, as hyperglycaemia will worsen ischaemic injury to the CNS. Hyperglycaemia causes anaerobic glycolysis, and the resultant lactic acidosis leads to deregulation of glucose metabolism, ionic homeostasis and free radical formation. There is no evidence that aggressive control of hyperglycaemia with insulin improves outcome. Hypoglycaemia must also be avoided, and glucose values maintained at between 4.0 and 10.0 mmol/l.

Colloids are useful when plasma volume expansion is required. Blood loss should be replaced with blood products as necessary. Blood flow through the cerebral microcirculation is improved if blood viscosity is reduced, and a haematocrit of 30 per cent is thought optimal.

Hypertonic solutions have been evaluated for use in resuscitation, as small volumes can produce rapid haemodynamic improvement. As hyperosmolality will reduce brain volume, these solutions may prove useful in the management of neurosurgical patients. Concerns about marked hypertonicity have prevented their widespread use.

Complications

Postoperative complications of neurosurgery are summarized in Box 10.1.

Fluid and electrolyte disturbances

Hyponatraemia

Hyponatraemia occurs relatively commonly in neurosurgical patients. It may be due to excess sodium loss, secondary to vomiting or diarrhoea, and administration of non-salt containing intravenous fluids. It may also develop following intracranial surgery

---

Box 10.1. Postoperative complications of neurosurgery

- Neurological deterioration – raised intracranial pressure; intracranial bleed
- Pain
- Nausea and vomiting
- Inappropriate antidiuretic hormone secretion (SIADH)
- Cerebal salt wasting syndrome
- Diabetes insipidus
- Seizures
- Vasospasm
- Thromboembolic complications

or subarachnoid haemorrhage (SAH) as a result of inappropriate antidiuretic hormone secretion (SIADH) or cerebral salt wasting (CSW). Although it can be difficult to distinguish between these two conditions, their treatments are very different.

- In SIADH, there is continued secretion of ADH despite a low plasma osmolality, resulting in water retention and hyponatraemia. The diagnosis is based on the finding of hyponatraemia with urinary sodium loss (>25 mmol/l). Treatment is aimed at fluid restriction, usually 500–1000 ml per day, depending on the sodium concentration. When fluid restriction is undesirable, demeclocycline (300–1200 mg/day) has been used successfully. Hypertonic saline solutions are rarely necessary unless the hyponatraemia is severe (<110 mmol/l).

- In CSW, there is a diuresis in addition to the natriuresis (urinary sodium >50 mmol/l), which may lead to a significant contraction of circulating and extracellular volumes. The pathology is unclear, although it may be related to secretion of a brain natriuretic peptide, an increase in atrial natriuretic peptide, or a defect in renal sodium reabsorption. In CSW syndrome, fluid restriction would not correct the hyponatraemia and may aggravate the hypovolaemia. Hypertonic fluid is used to correct the sodium deficit, and the sodium concentration should be increased gradually (~1 mmol/hr) to avoid the risk of central pontine myelinolysis.

Hypernatraemia
Hypernatraemia may occur as a result of excessive fluid restriction or aggressive osmotic therapy for ICP control. In these patients, hypernatraemia is treated with isotonic fluids. Diabetes insipidus is relatively common after pituitary or hypothalamic surgery, but it may also occur with other cerebral pathology (e.g. head injury or tumour). With the failure of ADH secretion the kidney is unable to conserve water, and large volumes of dilute urine are excreted. Diabetes insipidus is diagnosed by a high urinary output (>150 ml/hr) with low urine osmolality (50–100 mosm/kg) in the presence of an increased plasma osmolality (Box 10.2). Management requires careful monitoring of fluid input and output. The patient should receive maintenance fluids plus three-quarters of the previous hour's urine output. Fluid replacement is with 0.45 per cent sodium chloride solution. If urine output exceeds

---

Box 10.2. Diabetes insipidus

Diagnosis:

- Urine output >150 ml/hr
- Urine osmolality 50–150 mosm/kg
- Plasma osmolality >290 mosm/kg.

Treatment:

- 0.45 per cent sodium chloride, maintenance requirements
- Plus three-quarters of previous hour's output
- DDAVP 10–20 μg b.d nasally, or 0.5–2 μg i.v.

---

300 ml/h, then desmopressin (DDAVP) is given (10–20 μg b.d. nasally or 0.5–2 μg i.v.).

Seizures

Seizure activity results in irreversible cell damage, which is directly related to the duration of the seizure and is unrelated to any associated hypoxia or acidosis. Seizures may occur in any postoperative neurosurgical patient. Particular risk factors include those having temporal or parietal surgery, depressed skull fracture or penetrating brain injury. A correctable medical (hypoxia, electrolyte disturbances, infection) or surgical (intracerebral haematoma, cerebral oedema) cause should be sought. The place of prophylactic anticonvulsant therapy for 'at risk' patients is unclear; some centres prescribe it routinely. Phenytoin is the drug of choice, but it must be given in a sufficient dose to ensure therapeutic plasma values are achieved in the immediate postoperative period (i.v. loading dose 15 mg/kg over 1 hour, maintenance 3–4 mg/kg per day).

A rapidly acting intravenous drug such as diazepam (5 mg) is useful for the immediate treatment of convulsions (see Chapter 12).

Thromboembolic complications

Thromboembolic prophylaxis in neurosurgical patients has always been controversial. Neurosurgical patients fall into a high-risk category, but neurosurgeons worry about the risk of bleeding and the possibility of catastrophic haemorrhage if patients are given subcutaneous heparin. Recent work suggests that heparin started on the first postoperative day does not increase the incidence of haemorrhage. Non-pharmacological prophylaxis (graduated pressure stockings, pneumatic compression boots etc.) should also be used in the perioperative period.

Vasospasm

Vasospasm subsequent to SAH remains a major cause of morbidity in patients following cerebral aneurysm surgery. Permanent neurological deficit may develop if it is not treated aggressively. Treatment is with nimodipine and, if symptomatic vasospasm persists, by augmentation of cardiac output and blood pressure by volume expansion and inotropes. This is described in Chapter 4.

11

Traumatic brain injury

Head injury remains one of the most important causes of death and long-term disability in young adults, with approximately 1 million patients presenting to hospitals in the United Kingdom each year. In the 5–35 years age group, 15–20 per cent of all deaths are the result of head injuries. Head injuries are three times more likely to occur in men, although this sex difference is less marked in children. The mechanism of head injury varies with population group; road traffic accidents, sporting accidents and assaults are common causes of head injury in young men, whereas falls are more common in the elderly. Alcohol is an important contributory factor. The outlook for head-injured patients has improved considerably, mainly as a result of better care in the immediate post-injury period aimed at preventing secondary brain injury.

Primary brain injury

The primary brain injury describes the damage that occurs at the time of initial impact. It might therefore be preventable (e.g. by wearing seat belts or bicycle helmets), but is not treatable. The extent of damage will depend on the force applied to the brain, and may be focal or diffuse and associated with a skull fracture.

Focal injuries

Most brain injury occurs due to axonal shearing as a result of movement of the brain within the skull. In focal injury the damage is confined to a relatively localized area. Focal injuries include contusions, haemorrhage or haematoma, and because of their mass effect, may require urgent surgical intervention.

- *Contusions* usually occur on the summits of gyri as these bear the brunt of impact against the inside of the skull. The contusion may occur directly beneath the area of impact (*coup* contusion) or remote from the area of injury (*contrecoup* contusion). Contusions may be single or multiple. The neurological deficit depends on the severity of the injury, and can range from mild concussion to coma. If the contusion occurs in a sensory or motor area, it may produce a focal deficit.

• *Haemorrhages* – intracerebral haemorrhages are found in 15 per cent of fatal head injuries, and can occur in any location. Intraventricular and intracerebellar haemorrhages are associated with a very high mortality.

• *Extradural haematomas* are relatively uncommon, but are important because they can be rapidly fatal. The classical history is of a period with minimal clinical signs, the 'lucid period', followed several hours later by coma. Extradural haematomas usually result from a tear in a dural artery, often the middle meningeal artery, and in 85 per cent of patients are associated with a linear skull fracture over the parietal or temporal region. The injury to the underlying brain is relatively minor, and prognosis from extradural haematoma is excellent providing there is prompt surgical evacuation.

• *Subdural haematomas* are found in about 30 per cent of head injuries, and carry a worse prognosis than extradural haematomas, due to associated brain injury. They are associated with cortical lacerations or rupture of the bridging veins that extend from the dura to the cortex.

Diffuse injuries
Diffuse brain injury is produced by acceleration–deceleration forces, which result in shearing of nerve fibres and microvascular structures as the brain substance moves inside the cranium. The term 'diffuse axonal injury' is used to describe widespread lesions throughout the subcortical white matter and brainstem. This occurs in severe head injuries, and is followed by prolonged unconsciousness. With less violent axonal disruption there may be temporary loss of function rather than cell disruption, leading to concussion (a brief period of unconsciousness). Diffuse head injury is more common in children, seen in up to 20 per cent of those with severe head injury.

Skull fractures
Skull fractures are relatively common but do not in themselves cause disability. However, the presence of a skull fracture should suggest the possibility of associated brain injury or bleeding, and all patients must be admitted to hospital for observation. Skull

fractures are less common in children due to their more elastic bones.

Skull fractures occur at the point of impact, where the bone is deformed inwards. Fractures may be linear or, if bony fragments enter the cranium, depressed. Elevation is usually indicated if the fragment is depressed more than the thickness of the skull. A compound depressed fracture is associated with a full-thickness scalp laceration, and requires early surgical exploration and toilet. A base of skull fracture is classically diagnosed by the clinical findings of cerebral spinal fluid (CSF) leak from the ear, otorrhoea, positive Battle's sign (bruising in the mastoid region), a haemotympanum (blood behind the tympanic membrane) and racoon eyes (periorbital bruising).

Secondary brain injury

Following the primary brain injury the brain is rendered particularly susceptible to secondary insults. This secondary damage will not be confined to the area of primary injury but also occurs in the penumbral region. Secondary damage begins from the moment of impact, although it may not become apparent for some time. Many different factors are involved, but the most important are hypoxia, systemic hypotension and intracranial hypertension. The common mechanism by which these insults produce neuronal damage is cerebral ischaemia.

Neurological complications include:

- Changes in cerebral blood flow (CBF)
- Depression of cerebral metabolism
- Loss of autoregulation
- Intracranial hypertension
- Cerebral oedema.

Cerebral ischaemia results in a cascade of biochemical events and pathological reactions that cause neuronal death. This complicated process involves the accumulation of glutamate and excitatory amino acids, resulting in increased intracellular calcium, the generation of free radicals, and activation of inflammatory mediators. The cascade of ionic and metabolic events leads to vasodilatation and cellular dysfunction, resulting in cerebral oedema and loss of autoregulation.

There are changes in global and regional CBF. Initially there is a reduction in cerebral blood flow, but this is followed by hyperaemia.

Several days after the injury the CBF begins to fall again. Cerebral vasospasm may also occur as a result of the presence of extravasated subarachnoid blood. Cerebral metabolism is depressed proportionally to the depth of the coma. However, as normal flow/metabolism coupling is lost, cerebral blood flow to these areas is not reduced and relative hyperaemia occurs. The loss of autoregulation means that CBF will vary directly with CPP. Cerebral swelling produces an increase in the intracranial volume. Initially, there is little change in ICP due to compensatory mechanisms, but when these are exhausted the ICP will increase markedly with any further increase in intracerebral content. Other causes of raised intracranial pressure include cerebral hyperaemia, haematoma and CSF obstruction. In the presence of impaired autoregulation and increased ICP, a higher MAP is required to maintain cerebral perfusion. Data suggest that a CPP of at least 70 mmHg is needed.

The pathophysiological changes resulting from cerebral ischaemia cause systemic complications, which include:

- Hypoxaemia
- Hypotension
- Hypertension
- Tachycardia
- ECG abnormalities
- Pulmonary oedema.

Hypoxaemia may occur from airway obstruction, aspiration or central respiratory depression, and associated chest or abdominal injuries. Neurogenic pulmonary oedema is rare. Hypotension has been found in a third of patients in A&E departments, and may be due to systemic causes. It results in decreased cerebral perfusion. Hypertension, cardiac arrhythmias and ECG abnormalities result from intracranial hypertension and brainstem compression.

Management of head injury
Immediate management
The aim of immediate management is the prevention of secondary insults. Assessment and resuscitation should proceed simultaneously; the Advanced Trauma Life Support (ATLS) system provides useful guidelines for the initial resuscitation. Securing the airway, maintaining oxygenation and avoiding hypotension is crucial to outcome. Once the airway, respiratory system and cardiovascular systems have been stabilized, the neurological

---

Box 11.1. Indications for intubation and ventilation

Immediate:

- Coma (GCS $\leqslant$ 8)
- Inability to protect airway
- Hypoxaemia ($Pa0_2$ <9 kPa on air or <13 kPa on oxygen)
- Hypercarbia ($PaCO_2$ >6 kPa)
- Spontaneous hyperventilation ($PaCO_2$ <3.5 kPa)
- Respiratory arrhythmia
- Associated chest injury.

Prior to inter or intra-hospital transfer:

- Deteriorating consciousness level
- Potential airway compromise (e.g. bilateral fractured mandible, bleeding into mouth)
- Seizures.

---

assessment can proceed. An attempt should be made to determine the precise time and mechanism of impact, as there may be an associated pattern of injury.

Airway and breathing

Oxygen should be given routinely to all patients. Indications for intubation and ventilation are given in Box 11.1. Cervical spine injury will be present in a significant proportion of head injuries, and manual in-line stabilization during induction and intubation is essential. Patients should be assumed to have a full stomach and managed accordingly with a rapid sequence induction and cricoid pressure. Suxamethonium may produce a transient rise in ICP, but this is unimportant compared with securing the airway. An orogastric tube should be inserted. Gastric distension is common following severe trauma. Muscle relaxants, appropriate sedation and analgesia should be used, and the lungs ventilated to maintain a $Pa0_2$ >13 kPa and a $PaCO_2$ of 4.0–4.5 kPa. The choice of anaesthetic drugs should be influenced by the cardiovascular status of the patient.

Circulation

Intravenous access should be obtained during assessment of the circulation. A combination of hypotension and raised ICP will impair cerebral perfusion and result in cerebral ischaemia. There is unequivocal evidence that hypotension (systolic blood pressure of <80 mmHg) is associated with poor outcome, and this must be avoided at all times. Invasive arterial monitoring and central venous pressure monitoring should be considered at an early stage. Hypotension rarely occurs in the absence of additional injuries except in young children and the elderly, when blood loss from the scalp can be significant. Alternative sites of blood loss should be actively sought, such as thoracoabdominal injury, pelvic or long bone fractures. Fluid resuscitation usually begins with crystalloid solutions such as 0.9 per cent sodium chloride. Glucose-containing solutions are avoided, as hyperglycaemia has been linked to poor outcome. Colloids and blood products are used as indicated. After appropriate fluid resuscitation, inotropic drugs may be indicated to increase mean arterial pressure and maintain cerebral perfusion pressure.

Further management of head injury
Neurological assessment
Neurological assessment can be made clinically by use of the Glasgow Coma Scale (GCS). This should be recorded when the patient is first seen and repeated regularly, especially in the first couple of hours following injury, to detect any change in condition. The Glasgow Coma Sum Score (GCSS) is the sum of the scores for the three levels of assessment, and is used to classify head injury severity (Box 11.2).

Further assessment includes pupillary size and response to light or unequal motor responses. These may be helpful in localizing the injury.

Imaging
Multiply injured patients should have chest, cervical spine and pelvic X-rays. The indications for a CT scan are shown in Box 11.3.

Box 11.2. Glasgow Coma Sum Score (GCSS) and head injury severity	
Severe head injury	GCS ≤ 8
Moderate head injury	GCS 9–12
Mild head injury	GCS 13–15

Box 11.3. Indications for a CT scan

- Coma (GCSS ≤ 8), persisting after resuscitation
- Deteriorating level of consciousness or focal neurological deficit
- Skull fracture with any of:
  - altered conscious level, seizures, neurological signs
- Open injury:
  - depressed skull fracture
  - basal skull
  - fracture penetrating injury.

Neurosurgical referral

The Royal College of Surgeons published a report on the management of head injuries in June 1999, and this makes several key recommendations regarding how these patients should then be managed. Patients with severe head injuries should be transferred to a specialist neurosurgical centre following initial assessment and resuscitation. Indications for referral to a neurosurgical unit are listed in Box 11.4.

Transfer of head injury patients

The transfer of patients is associated with risks, and inevitably leads to delay in neurosurgical intervention. However, the increase in mortality associated with patient transfer is not attributable to

---

Box 11.4. Indications for referral to a neurosurgical unit

Immediately after initial assessment and resuscitation:
- Coma (GCSS ≤ 8), persisting after resuscitation
- Deteriorating level of consciousness or focal neurological deficits
- Skull fracture with any of:
  - altered conscious level
  - seizures
  - neurological symptoms or signs.

Urgently:
- Open injury:
  - depressed skull fracture
  - basal skull fracture
  - penetrating injury
- Confusion or neurological disturbance for more than 6 hours
- Persistent or worsening headache or vomiting.

Box 11.5. Guidelines for transfer of patients with acute head injury

---

- Thorough resuscitation and stabilization of the patient should be achieved before transfer
- All patients with severe head injury should be sedated, intubated and ventilated, except in exceptional circumstances
- Adequate equipment and monitoring should be available, and monitoring during transfer should be of a standard appropriate to a patient needing intensive care
- Local guidelines, consistent with established national guidelines, should exist and be known by the staff involved
- A doctor with at least 2 years experience in the appropriate specialty should accompany the patient, and trained assistance should be available
- The ability to communicate with both the base hospital and the receiving centre should exist in case problems arise *en route*.

---

transfer time or distance, but to suboptimal care during transfer. The document *Recommendations for the Transfer of Patients with Acute Head injuries to Neurosurgical Units* (published by the Neuroanaesthesia Society and the Association of Anaesthetists of Great Britain & Ireland) provides guidelines, and these are outlined in Box 11.5.

Management in intensive care

Intensive care management of head injury is aimed at providing optimal cerebral oxygenation by the maintenance of cerebral perfusion. Complications such as hypotension, hypoxia, raised intracranial pressure, reduced cerebral perfusion pressure and pyrexia, which have been found to contribute to poor outcome, should be identified and treated promptly.

Principles of management

All patients with severe head injury should be sedated, intubated and ventilated. Arterial oxygen saturation should be optimal and patients ventilated to maintain $PaCO_2$ ~4.5 kPa. Patients should be nursed with the head position neutral and a slight 15–30° head-up tilt. Sedation and analgesia should be adequate and reassessed regularly. Additional boluses may be necessary before interventions that might increase ICP.

Cerebral metabolic demands should be kept to a minimum, as

Box 11.6. Management principles for acute head injury

- Clear airway
- Adequate ventilation and oxygenation
- Avoidance of hypotension
- Control of ICP.

---

increases in cerebral oxygen consumption may increase cerebral ischaemia. Hyperpyrexia and seizures should be avoided. Continuous EEG monitoring is useful in sedated and paralysed patients. Prophylactic anticonvulsants may reduce the incidence of early seizures.

ICP monitoring enables the calculation of CPP, and maintenance of a CPP >70 mmHg is associated with a better outcome following head injury. Arterial pressure should be maintained with appropriate intravenous fluids. Glucose-containing solutions are avoided because of the risk of hyperglycaemia worsening ischaemic cerebral damage. An insulin infusion may be necessary to maintain normoglycaemia. Inotropic drugs may be indicated, especially in the presence of a high ICP when an increased MAP is needed to achieve the desired CPP.

The principles of management for acute head injury are summarized in Box 11.6.

Management of intracranial pressure

Raised ICP pressure is associated with an increased morbidity and mortality after head injury. Intracranial hypertension may be due to cerebral oedema, increased cerebral blood flow, intracranial haematoma or acute hydrocephalus. Clinical signs are late and inconsistent; hence the need for ICP monitoring in all patients with severe head injury. Continuous monitoring of ICP allows early detection of adverse events and assessment of the efficacy of therapeutic interventions.

Attention to the general principles discussed above, and correction of any remediable causes (Box 11.7), should take priority before the implementation of specific therapies for the treatment of intracranial hypertension.

Specific therapies
- Mannitol 0.25–0.5 g/kg over 15 minutes will decrease ICP if used appropriately (intermittent boluses, titrated against ICP)

Box 11.7. Remediable causes of raised ICP

- Inadequate ventilation: hypoxia or hypercapnia
- Airway obstruction
- Hypotension/hypertension
- Poor patient positioning – neck flexion or rotation
- Inadequate sedation/analgesia/neuromuscular blockade
- Coughing or straining
- Pyrexia
- Seizures.

- Hyperventilate patient to $PaCO_2$ of about 3.5 kPa; the effect is only temporary
- Increase MAP with intravenous fluids or inotropic drugs to raise CPP
- Drain CSF via an external ventricular catheter
- Trial with a bolus of intravenous anaesthetic agent such as thiopentone or propofol; if successful, use an infusion
- Hypothermia
- Surgical decompression.

Cerebral protection

There is increasing evidence to support moderate hypothermia (34–36°C) in head injury to reduce cerebral oxygen consumption and hence provide neuroprotection. Pyrexia increases $CMRO_2$, and should be avoided at all costs. Metabolic suppressant agents such as barbiturates may be useful in certain patients with intractable intracranial hypertension, when titrated to produce burst suppression on the EEG. However, they prolong recovery and result in cardiovascular depression. Other neuroprotective agents, such as excitatory amino acid antagonists, antioxidants and calcium channel blockers, are at present experimental.

Outcome

Assessment of outcome can be made using the Glasgow Outcome Score (see Box 11.8).

Various factors have an adverse effect on outcome, including:

- Age – this seems to be the most important patient-dependent factor; the elderly have a higher mortality, independent of pre-existing disease

---

Box 11.8. Glasgow Outcome Score (GOS)

1 Death
2 Persistent vegetative state
3 Severe disability (conscious but disabled)
4 Moderate disability (disabled but independent)
5 Good recovery.

- Mechanism of injury and intracranial pathology – patients with mass lesions have a higher mortality than those with a diffuse injury; penetrating injuries have a higher mortality for the same GCSS
- Intracranial hypertension
- Hypotension
- Secondary insults.

The time of assessment must be stated.

Neurological intensive care

There are three main groups of patients encountered on the neurointensive care unit; those with:

1 *Intracranial lesions* – these may be the result of trauma, haemorrhage, tumour, or infarction
2 *Respiratory depression* – those with (or at risk of) acute respiratory depression as a result of a peripheral nervous system disorder affecting the nerves, the neuromuscular junction or the muscles, or as the result of a CNS disorder such as status epilepticus, cerebral ischaemia or coma
3 *CNS infections* – infections such as meningitis, encephalitis and brain abscess.

Patients with intracranial lesions make up the majority of patients admitted to the neurointensive care unit, and their management is discussed in other chapters. The other groups of patients are dealt with here, together with the diagnosis of brain death and the management of the brain dead patient.

Peripheral nervous system disorders

The major problem in patients with neuromuscular disease is weakness, and this can be life threatening when it affects the bulbar or respiratory muscles. Respiratory failure may develop in many of these conditions, but those most frequently encountered on the intensive care unit are Guillain–Barré syndrome and myasthenia gravis. Before the successful vaccination programme, poliomyelitis was the most common peripheral nervous system disorder requiring ventilatory support. It is now rarely seen, but still remains a problem in the developing world.

Guillain–Barré syndrome

Guillain–Barré syndrome is the name given to a group of acute inflammatory demyelinating polyneuropathies. It is the most common peripheral nervous system disorder requiring ventilatory support. It has an incidence of one to two cases per 100 000 population and can occur at any age. In more than 60 per cent of patients there is a history of a preceding flu-like illness, and there is evidence for the involvement of cytomegalovirus, Epstein–Barr virus, *Campylobacter jejuni* and *Mycoplasma pneumoniae* in the pathogenesis. Surgery and immunization have also been implicated in the development of the syndrome.

Clinical features
Initial presentation is usually with muscle weakness starting in the legs and ascending at a variable rate. Weakness tends to be symmetrical, and may have been preceded by paraesthesiae in the hands and feet. Cranial nerve involvement, typically of the facial and bulbar nerves, is found in up to 50 per cent of patients. Back pain may be a presenting feature, and is often severe. As the condition progresses, neuropathic pain becomes more of a feature and may be difficult to treat. Respiratory muscle weakness combined with the inability to clear secretions results in the need for ventilatory support. Motor reflexes are absent. Sensory loss is generally mild. Autonomic dysfunction is present in 65 per cent of patients, and may result in postural hypotension, dysrrhythmias and cardiovascular instability. Persistent hyponatraemia may occur as a result of the syndrome of inappropriate ADH secretion.

The natural history of the condition is variable. There is usually a period of progression lasting between 1 and 3 weeks, followed by a plateau phase lasting for 2–4 weeks and then slow improvement.

Investigations
Diagnosis is based on the history plus the findings of raised CSF protein (>0.4 g/l) and a normal white cell count ($< 10^3$/l). Nerve conduction studies show delayed conduction as a result of demyelination.

Management
Management is directed at specific treatment of the condition itself and general supportive therapy. Specific treatments include:

• Plasma exchange. This has been shown to be effective; it accelerates recovery and shortens the duration of ventilatory support.

The volume of plasma exchange varies from 50 to 200 ml/kg on three to five occasions.

- Intravenous immunoglobulins. These have been shown to be equally effective and may be better tolerated in unstable patients. An infusion of 0.4 mg/kg is given daily over a 5-day period. As with plasma exchange, despite reducing the duration of disability, intravenous immunoglobulins do not decrease mortality. Intravenous immunoglobulins are easier to administer than plasma exchange, but they are expensive and not without risks; both anaphylaxis and renal failure have been reported.
- Steroids. However, there is no evidence that these are effective.

General therapy is supportive, and focuses on:

- Respiratory support. This is needed in up to 33 per cent of patients and should be anticipated. Clinical assessment and measurement of vital capacity are most helpful. This should be carried out at least twice a day while the condition is progressing. Arterial blood gas analysis is of little use. Indications for intubation and ventilation are listed in Box 12.1. Suxamethonium should be avoided because of its effects on the denervated muscle and the risk of hyperkalaemia. As mechanical ventilation is often needed for several weeks, early tracheostomy is usually recommended.
- Cardiovascular support. This may be necessary in those patients with an autonomic neuropathy. Hypotension may occur on starting pulmonary ventilation. Pacemaker insertion may be needed.
- Nutritional support. Nasogastric feeding should be instituted unless there is an ileus, when parenteral nutrition may be necessary.
- Analgesia. This is needed in the majority of patients. Pain is often resistant to simple analgesics and opiates. Antidepressants, anticonvulsants and epidural opioids have all been used with success.
- Psychological support. This is invariably needed. Many patients are terrified and believe that they are dying. Constant reassurance

---

Box 12.1. Indications for intubation and ventilation in Guillain–Barré syndrome

- Vital capacity <15 ml/kg or <50 per cent predicted
- Respiratory rate >30/min
- Inadequate cough.

and support from the medical team is very important, and anxio-
lytics or antidepressants may be helpful.
- Thromboembolic prophylaxis. This should be instituted.
- Physiotherapy for the chest and passive movements for the limbs.
This is essential to prevent contracture formation.

Outcome
With advances in supportive therapy the mortality rate from
Guillain–Barré has dropped dramatically to about 5 per cent.
Full recovery usually takes months. About 25 per cent of patients
may still not have fully recovered at 1 year, and a significant proportion of these may be left with a permanent deficit. In patients
who develop a chronic relapsing form of Guillain–Barré the diagnosis of chronic demyelinating inflammatory polyneuropathy
should be considered. This seems to be a distinct condition, and
may respond to steroids.

Myasthenia gravis
Myasthenia gravis is an autoimmune disorder of neuromuscular
transmission characterized by muscle weakness and fatiguability
on sustained effort. The incidence is about one to five in 100 000,
and it is more common in women. It may occur at any age, but has
two peaks: in women at 20–30 years and in men at 50–60 years.

Pathophysiology
The main findings are a simplification of the post-junctional membrane with a reduction in the number of acetylcholine receptors
(ACh-Rs) and the presence of IgG antibodies against the ACh-
Rs. The production of these antibodies is T cell dependent. There
is often an associated thymoma (10–15 per cent) or, more commonly, thymic hyperplasia (65 per cent).

Clinical features
Symptoms are of increasing muscle weakness, worse as the day
progresses and following exercise. Typically the weakness improves
after rest. Striated muscles in any part of the body may be affected,
often asymmetrically. However, weakness of the muscles of the eyes
and face, giving rise to diplopia and ptosis, is the most common
initial presentation. If the symptoms do not progress, the diagnosis
is that of ocular myasthenia gravis. However, most patients (80
per cent) develop additional muscle weakness. The facial, neck,

limb and respiratory muscles all may be involved. The proximal muscles of the upper limbs are affected more frequently than those of the lower limbs. Bulbar palsy may produce difficulties with swallowing and speech. The severity and natural history of myasthenia gravis are highly variable and unpredictable.

Investigation

Diagnosis is confirmed by demonstrating an improvement in symptoms in response to edrophonium (2–10 mg i.v.). Improvement should be seen within about 5 minutes and last for 30–60 minutes. The test is not specific, and false positives may occur in other conditions. ACh-R antibodies are present in about 80–90 per cent of patients with generalized myasthenia gravis, and there is a decremental response to repeated nerve stimulation on electromyography. All patients with myasthenia gravis should have a CT scan of the chest to exclude a thymoma.

Management

- *Anticholinesterase drugs*. Pyridostigmine and neostigmine provide symptomatic treatment. Pyridostigmine tends to be the most frequently used because it has a longer duration of action and fewer muscarinic side effects, but concurrent treatment with anticholinergic drugs may be required.
- *Thymectomy*. This is beneficial in nearly all patients. It is indicated in all patients with a thymoma, and is increasingly advocated in all patients. It appears especially beneficial in young women with thymic hyperplasia.
- *Corticosteroids*. These are effective in 70 per cent of patients, and seem particularly effective in older patients. Initial high-dose treatment seems to give the best results, but occasionally patients may experience transient exacerbation of their symptoms.
- *Immunosuppressants*. Agents such as azathioprine and cyclophosphamide seem to be effective adjuncts to steroid therapy, but may lead to neutropenia and infection.
- *Plasma exchange*. This seems to be an effective short-term treatment for severe exacerbations, and various regimens have been suggested.
- *Intravenous immunoglobulins*. Immunoglobulins have also been used with success in acute crises.

Intensive care management
Intensive care is most commonly required for postoperative care following thymectomy or for the management of respiratory failure, which is usually the result of a crisis.

• A myasthenic crisis is a life-threatening deterioration in a patient with myasthenia gravis. It may be precipitated by infection, surgery or certain drugs (see Box 12.2), and a precipitating cause should be sought and treated. Crises occur in up to 20 per cent of patients with myasthenia gravis, and usually happen in the first 2 years following diagnosis.

• A cholinergic crisis may also cause rapid deterioration, but occurs as a consequence of excess anticholinesterase drugs. A cholinergic crisis should be distinguishable clinically from a myasthenic crisis by the associated muscarinic effects (abdominal colic, diarrhoea, sweating and bradycardia); however, in practice it may be difficult to distinguish between the two. In a cholinergic crisis, anticholinesterase drugs are withheld and the patient should improve. If the diagnosis is in doubt, edrophonium 2–10 mg i.v. may be given. If following edrophonium the condition deteriorates the diagnosis is that of a cholinergic crisis, but if it improves it is a myasthenic crisis.

During a crisis, intensive care admission is essential. Intubation and ventilation should be considered in any patient with a bulbar palsy or a vital capacity <15 ml/kg, and for exhaustion. Anticholinesterase drugs are usually withheld for several days after intubation to reduce airway secretions. High-dose steroids and plasma exchange should be started simultaneously, and improvement may be noticed

---

Box 12.2. Drugs that may exacerbate a myasthenic crisis

• Antibiotics: aminoglycosides, penicillins, sulphonamides, polymyxin, fluoroquinolones, tetracycline
• Antiarrhythmics: quinine, quinidine, procainamide, beta-blockers, calcium channel antagonists
• Local anaesthetics: lignocaine
• Muscle relaxants
• Lithium
• Phenothiazines
• Anti-spasmodics: baclofen, benzodiazepines
• Anti-rheumatoid drugs.

within a few days. Ventilation is rarely prolonged, and in the absence of other complications tracheostomy is unnecessary. Intensive care management is otherwise supportive, providing nutrition, physiotherapy etc.

Myasthenic syndromes

Eaton–Lambert syndrome is also an autoimmune disorder affecting neuromuscular transmission. There are autoantibodies to voltage-gated calcium channels in the presynaptic membrane leading to a reduction in ACh release. It was originally described in association with small cell carcinoma of the lung, but also occurs without an associated malignancy.

Muscle weakness tends to be most pronounced in the proximal limbs and, although the patient may complain of fatiguability, muscle weakness tends to decrease following exercise. Other neurological features are reduced or absent tendon reflexes, autonomic involvement and ptosis. Respiratory failure is rare. Electromyography (EMG) shows a decrease in amplitude of the EMG muscle potential. However, with higher frequency stimulation, or following muscle contraction, there is an increase in amplitude. Diagnosis may be confirmed by the presence of antibodies.

Treatment requires removal (if possible) of the underlying malignancy, improvement of neuromuscular transmission, and immunosuppression. Improvement has been seen with 3,4-diaminopyridine, which increases the release of ACh. Corticosteroids and plasma exchange are also effective.

Central nervous system disorders

Central nervous system disorders affecting the respiratory centres in the brainstem often result in respiratory failure, but respiratory depression is a frequent accompaniment of any CNS disorder that produces altered consciousness. Cerebral vascular disease or stroke is the most common neurological disease requiring hospital admission. However, patients with ischaemic stroke rarely require intensive care admission. The management of patients with subarachnoid haemorrhage is covered elsewhere.

Status epilepticus is one of the commonest neurological emergencies, and frequently requires admission to the intensive care unit.

Status epilepticus

Epilepsy is a common condition (incidence 0.5–1 per cent), and of these patients up to 5 per cent will develop status epilepticus. Seizure activity also occurs in up to 10 per cent of patients on a general ITU, and may occur in any postoperative neurosurgical patient. Status epilepticus is a single seizure, prolonged for more than 30 minutes, or sequential seizures occurring without full recovery between them. It is a medical emergency – the associated mortality is about 10 per cent – and requires prompt intervention. Prolonged seizure activity results in neuronal necrosis, and the extent of this is directly related to the duration of the seizure.

Pathophysiology

Epilepsy should be thought of as a symptom rather than a diagnosis. Status epilepticus can occur in an established epileptic as a result of a change in antiepileptic medication, poor compliance, drug interactions or intercurrent illnesses. It may also occur as a presenting symptom, and a precipitating or underlying cause should always be sought (see Box 12.3). There is a much greater likelihood of an acute brain abnormality or an underlying metabolic disturbance in adults.

At a cellular level, metabolic demands in continuously firing neurones increase by 200–300 per cent, resulting in hypoxia and ischaemia. Neuronal necrosis occurs as a result of accumulation of excitatory neurotransmitters. This damage is exacerbated by the associated systemic changes, such as tachycardia, hypertension and hypoglycaemia. A consequence of the increased muscle activity, which occurs in prolonged seizures, is increased production of carbon dioxide and inadequate ventilation. The result is a mixed

---

Box 12.3. Causes of seizures in the intensive care unit

- Cerebrovascular events – intracerebral bleed, cerebral infarction, SAH
- Encephalopathies
- Infection – meningitis
- Hypoxia
- Sepsis
- Mass lesions
- Drug toxicity/withdrawal
- Renal/hepatic dysfunction.

respiratory and metabolic acidosis, hypoxia and hyperthermia. The longer the seizure activity continues the more likely it is that decompensation will occur, with irreversible brain damage, rhabdomyolysis, renal failure, cardiovascular collapse and, eventually, death.

Investigations
A list of investigations is detailed below, but history and clinical findings may point to specific or additional investigations.

- Full blood count, urea and electrolytes, glucose, liver function tests and calcium
- Arterial blood gases
- Drug levels of antiepileptics
- Toxicology screen
- Urinalysis
- Lumbar puncture to exclude CNS infection (if there is no evidence of raised intracranial pressure)
- CT/MRI – most patients with status epilepticus should have neuroimaging unless they have been thoroughly investigated in the past; MRI is more useful than CT
- EEG – this can be of particular value in distinguishing psychogenic status and in diagnosing non-convulsive status
- ICP.

Management
Assessment, investigations and treatment should proceed simultaneously. Priorities include management of the airway, breathing and circulation, and prompt control of the seizures.

- ABC – secure airway, give oxygen, obtain venous access and stabilize vital signs.
- Benzodiazepines are the commonest first-line drugs, but respiratory depression should be watched for:
  - Diazepam i.v. 2–5 mg bolus, repeated each minute until seizures stop, to a total of 20 mg
  - Clonazepam i.v. 0.25–0.5 mg bolus, repeated each minute until seizures stop, to a total of 5 mg
  - Lorazepam i.v. 4 mg bolus, repeated after 20 minutes if there is no effect.

- Give phenytoin to prevent recurrence of the seizures – 15 mg/kg as a loading dose, slowly (not more than 50 mg per minute). Cardiac arrhythmias and hypotension may occur.
- Correct hypoglycaemia. If the patient is hypoglycaemic, 1 ml/kg of 50 per cent glucose should be given.
- Correct treatable cause – e.g. meningitis, raised intracranial pressure, hyponatraemia.
- Stop seizures. Give thiopentone or propofol infusions if fits are not controlled after 60 minutes. The objective is to produce burst suppression on the EEG. This may be difficult to achieve, but may not be essential as long as the epileptiform EEG activity ceases.
- Management of systemic complications. If large doses of anticonvulsants are required, or the level of consciousness is depressed, intubation and ventilation will be required. Cardiovascular support should be provided as indicated. Hyperthermia, acidosis, rhabdomyolysis and cerebral oedema should be treated.
- Alternative drugs:

  - Chlormethiazole is given as an intravenous infusion, 0.8 per cent solution, 15 ml/min up to 100 ml, then reduced and titrated against seizure activity; it is initially rapidly cleared from the circulation, but accumulates if continued for any length of time
  - Phenobarbitone 10–15 mg/kg i.v. slowly
  - Paraldehyde 0.2 ml/kg diluted with normal saline, either i.m. or p.r.

Box 12.4. Management of status epilepticus

- ABC. Secure airway, give oxygen, obtain venous access and stabilize vital signs
- Give diazepam 20 mg i.v. over 5 minutes; repeat if necessary
- Give phenytoin 15 mg/kg i.v. to prevent recurrence of the seizures
- Correct treatable causes, such as hypoglycaemia.

If control is not achieved, consider:

- Chlormethiazole 0.8 per cent solution – 15 ml/min up to 100 ml, then reduced and titrated against seizure activity; or phenobarbitone 10–15 mg/kg i.v.
- For refractory seizures, thiopentone or propofol.

Outcome
Mortality is related to the underlying CNS or systemic disease causing the status epilepticus. Mortality increases with age, and is also linked to the duration of the status. If the seizures have not been controlled within 12 hours, mortality rates greater than 80 per cent have been reported.

Cerebral ischaemia

Although ischaemic cerebral vascular disease is the third most common cause of death in the western world and the most common neurological disease process requiring hospitalization, patients are rarely admitted to the intensive care unit. However, this may be necessary when there is loss of consciousness or respiratory failure. In brainstem strokes, the respiratory centres themselves may be affected. In cortical strokes, cerebral oedema and raised intracranial pressure result in brainstem dysfunction and respiratory depression. Most deaths occurring in the first few days are the direct consequence of the brain damage, but subsequent deaths are usually the result of systemic complications such as pneumonia, pulmonary embolus, myocardial infarction and infections.

Pathophysiology
The term 'stroke' is applied to a clinical syndrome lasting more than 24 hours in which an acute, focal cerebral deficit occurs secondary to cerebrovascular disease. If symptoms resolve within 24 hours it is termed a transient ischaemic attack (TIA). Of those admitted with permanent neurological deficit, about 80 per cent will be due to cerebral infarction and up to 20 per cent due to cerebral haemorrhage. Cerebral infarction may be due to thrombotic occlusion of vessels (two-thirds) or emboli (one-third). Thrombotic strokes are more common in patients with hypertension, hypercholesterolaemia, diabetes etc. Embolic strokes occur in patients with underlying cardiac disease such as atrial fibrillation, valvular disease or myocardial infarction. In younger patients, ischaemic strokes may occur as a result of vasculitis or disorders of coagulation.

Investigations
These will be based on the clinical history and examination, and should help to determine the type of stroke, its likely cause, and the development of complications. Investigations include:

- Full blood count, urea, electrolytes, creatinine, glucose
- Detailed coagulation screen
- Serum lipid profile (these are unreliable in the acute setting)
- ECG – to detect cardiac arrhythmias, myocardial infarction
- CT scan or MRI – this should be performed as soon as possible to help distinguish cerebral haemorrhage from infarction
- Angiography – if an underlying vascular malformation is suspected
- Echocardiogram – if a cardioembolic stroke is thought likely
- Carotid dopplers or transcranial doppler.

Management
The decision as whether to admit these patients to the intensive care unit must be made on an individual basis, but it has been estimated that about 10 per cent of stroke patients might benefit. Intensive care management is largely supportive, aiming at control of blood pressure, providing respiratory support, nutritional care, and intracranial pressure management. There is still no proven specific treatment for stroke, although thrombolytic agents seem promising:

- Aspirin 160–300mg. This may be beneficial, and is given as soon as possible after acute ischaemic stroke.
- Thrombolysis. The potential benefits of thrombolysis are clot lysis and reperfusion, but there is an associated risk of haemorrhage. Several large, randomized controlled trials have been undertaken, but unfortunately the results so far have not been conclusive. In patients with cardioembolic strokes anticoagulation is beneficial, but should be withheld until CT scan is performed and shows that there is no haemorrhage present.
- Neuroprotective agents – so far results have been disappointing.

Metabolic encephalopathy
Metabolic encephalopathies almost always present with an increasing confusional state or delirium, which may progress to coma. There are many causes (see Box 12.5). The most common are metabolic and pharmacological, but diagnosis may be difficult.

Investigation
This should start with a complete medical history and a thorough examination. Laboratory tests can then be based on these findings, but might include:

Box 12.5. Causes of metabolic encephalopathies

- Hepatic encephalopathy
- Uraemic encephalopathy
- Electrolyte disturbances
- Hyper- or hypo-osmolar states
- Hypo- or hyperglycaemia
- Drug intoxication.

- Urinalysis – for glucose, ketones
- Full blood count and examination of blood film
- Urea, electrolytes, creatinine and glucose
- Toxicology screen
- Endocrine – specific hormone assays, if thought appropriate from history and examination
- CT scan or MRI
- LP – if CNS infection is suspected and there is not raised ICP
- EEG.

Management
Management will depend on the underlying cause. Any reversible pathology must be corrected immediately. Priorities are management of airway, breathing and circulation. Neurological assessment should detect and intervene in the event of any deterioration. Additional intensive care is aimed at preventing complications.

Outcome
The prognosis depends on the underlying cause of the coma and its duration.

Central nervous system infections
Central nervous system infections requiring admission to the intensive care unit are meningitis, encephalitis and cerebral abscess.

Meningitis
Acute bacterial meningitis is a medical emergency. Mortality rates vary with the infecting organism, the age and underlying medical condition of the patient. In addition, the earlier the diagnosis is made and the sooner treatment is started, the better the survival rates.

Pathophysiology
The pathogenesis of the events leading to death and neurological sequelae are complex. Bacterial antigens initiate the production of inflammatory mediators such as complement and cytokines, including tumour necrosis factor (TNF) and interleukin-1β, which in turn induce the formation of selectins and integrins. This inflammatory process disrupts the blood–brain barrier and produces the typical changes of acute meningeal inflammation and purulent exudate in the subarachnoid space. These events lead to cerebral oedema, obstruction to CSF pathways and raised intracranial pressure.

The causative organism is age related, but the commonest include *Haemophilus influenzae, Streptococcus pneumoniae* and *Neisseria meningitidis*. In neonates, the most common organisms are group B streptococci and gram-negative enterobacteria. In children, the most common organisms are *H. influenzae* and *N. meningitidis*. Meningococcal meningitis is most often seen in children and adolescents, and pneumococcal meningitis in adults. There has been a dramatic reduction in the incidence of meningitis caused by meningococcus C and *H. influenzae* as a result of immunization programmes.

Clinical features
Clinical features of bacterial meningitis include severe headache, neck stiffness, photophobia, pyrexia and impaired consciousness level (meningism). A petechial rash suggests the possibility of meningoccal septicaemia, but can occur with other organisms. Circulatory collapse may occur with meningoccal septicaemia.

Chronic meningitis differs in that it usually develops slowly over weeks or months. Presentation is with headache, malaise, confusion, cranial nerve palsies or seizures. The most common organism is tuberculosis, but other organisms such as mycoplasmas, legionellas and fungi can occur.

Investigations
Diagnosis is based on the clinical picture plus the presence of white blood cells, predominantly polymorphonuclear pleocytosis, along with microorganisms in the CSF.

Management
Management is based on early diagnosis, appropriate antibiotic regimens, and treating complications. Steroids have been shown

to reduce the incidence of neurological sequelae in children. Intensive care is needed in patients with significantly depressed consciousness level or for cardiovascular support.

Outcome
Advances in antibiotic regimens, immunization and intensive care have led to a marked reduction in mortality, but it is still high at 15 per cent. Neurological complications are also significant, with behavioural problems, sensorineural deafness, cognitive defects and visual disturbances occurring in 20–50 per cent of children.

Encephalitis
The most common encephalitis seen on the neurointensive care unit is herpes simplex encephalitis. It has an incidence of about one per 250 000 per annum, and is still associated with a high mortality despite advances in treatment.

Pathophysiology
Pathological changes are inflammation with haemorrhagic congestion and gliosis. It is not associated with immunosuppression. Infection spreads along the olfactory nerve to the temporal lobe, insular and cingulate gyrus and frontal cortex.

Clinical features
The clinical picture is of pyrexia, confusion, personality change, deteriorating consciousness level and seizures. It has usually been preceded by a short prodromal illness with headache and fever. In the majority of patients it is reactivation of an existing infection. Patients are often critically ill, with impaired consciousness and raised ICP. Seizures can be difficult to control.

Investigations
Diagnosis is based on the clinical picture with the detection of virus specific antibodies in the blood and CSF. There are EEG changes typical of herpes simplex encephalitis, with spike and slow wave activity associated with periodic complexes. Abnormalities may be seen in the temporal lobes on CT scan or MRI.

Management
Treatment is with acyclovir, which should be started as soon as the diagnosis is suspected. These patients are often critically ill and

require intensive care management for cardiorespiratory support and control of seizures.

Outcome

Mortality has been reduced to 20 per cent, but many survivors are left with complications. The earlier treatment is instigated, the better the outcome.

Cerebral abscesses

Cerebral abscesses occur less commonly than meningitis.

Pathophysiology

Cerebral abscesses may occur as a result of direct extension of local infection – for example, secondary to middle ear or sinus infections, or as a result of penetrating trauma, either accidental or operative. Alternatively, spread may be from a distant site such as bacterial endocarditis, when the abscesses may be multiple. The causative organisms will be related to the initial site of infection. Middle ear and dental infections are often anaerobic. Sinus infections are usually Staphylococcus aureus, Haemophilus influenzae or Streptoccus pneumoniae. In the immunocompromised patient, Toxoplasma, Aspergillus, Listeria and Candida may be found.

Clinical features

Symptoms relate to the size and location of the abscess. They include signs of raised ICP, such as headache, nausea and vomiting, or patients may present with focal neurological deficits, indistinguishable from those caused by any other space-occupying lesion but more rapidly progressive. Pyrexia is not usually a significant feature.

Investigations

Diagnosis is made on CT or MRI findings, and from organisms isolated either from the lesion itself or blood cultures. Often these patients have a known clinical diagnosis that puts them at risk of a cerebral abscess. Since the advent of stereotactic techniques, aspiration of cerebral abscesses can be performed quickly and safely.

Management

Treatment is three-fold: surgical aspiration, appropriate antibiotic therapy and treatment of the primary source of infection.

Outcome
Mortality is around 10 per cent, but is dependent on prompt diagnosis and treatment of the underlying pathology. Epilepsy is the most common complication.

Brain death

As a consequence of advances in intensive care, cardiorespiratory function can be sustained for days in the presence of total and irreversible brain damage. Brain death refers to the permanent cessation of neuronal function in the whole brain, including the cerebral hemispheres, the brainstem and the cerebellum. However, it is now generally accepted that when the brainstem is dead the brain is dead, and that this equates with clinical death. The majority of the medical profession and the general public accept this concept of brain death. To prolong mechanical ventilation in these circumstances is not only futile but also causes unnecessary suffering to the patient and relatives. The time of death is, therefore, the time when brain death is diagnosed; not some time later when the heart stops.

However, the diagnosis must be made with absolute certainty because of the enormity of its implications. Not only is it the basis for withdrawing treatment, but also consent may then be obtained for the brain-dead patient to become an organ donor. Hence, the Royal Colleges and their Faculties established criteria for brainstem death in 1976. Since then, different countries and institutions have developed their own sets of criteria. In the United Kingdom a revised Code of Practice was published in 1998, and current practice is based on this document.

The diagnosis of brain death is a three-part process. Before formal testing can be carried out, each of the first two parts must be satisfied.

1 Preconditions for brain death:
  • The patient's condition is due to irreversible brain damage, the cause of which is known
  • The patient is in unresponsive coma.
2 Exclusions – the exclusion of other, potentially reversible causes of brainstem depression:
  • Pharmacological causes – narcotics, alcohol, residual effects of sedatives or neuromuscular agents

---

Box 12.6. Brain death – brainstem reflexes

- No pupillary response to light: the pupils do not respond either directly or consensually to sharp changes in the intensity of light
- Absent corneal reflex: no response to direct stimulation of the cornea
- Absent vestibulo-ocular reflex: no eye movements following slow injection of 50 ml ice-cold water into each auditory meatus in turn
- No motor response to central stimulation: no motor response within the cranial nerve distribution in response to a sustained painful stimulus
- Absent gag reflex: no contraction of the soft palate when the uvula is stimulated
- Absent cough reflex: no response to bronchial stimulation by a catheter passed through the endotracheal tube.

- Metabolic disorders and endocrine disorders; hypernatraemia is a frequent finding in brain dead patients and does not in itself preclude the diagnosis
- Hypothermia.

If there are any doubts about the primary diagnosis, then do not proceed.

3 Clinical tests. These may only be performed if the preconditions and exclusions are satisfied. They must be performed by two doctors, one a consultant and the other at least a senior registrar with 5 years' post-qualification. If organ donation is a possibility, neither doctor should have any connection with the transplant team. The tests should be repeated to exclude observer error. Testing involves confirmation of the absence of brainstem reflexes (Box 12.6) and the absence of spontaneous respiration (Box 12.7).

If the patient has chronic obstructive pulmonary disease and is insensitive to hypercapnia, relying on the hypoxic drive to breathe, a 'normal' set of arterial blood gases for that patient should be obtained during disconnection, and the $PaCO_2$ allowed to fall by a further 1–2 kPa. If there is any doubt about the ability to provide adequate stimulus, then the patient is not suitable for testing.

Following the two sets of tests, the patient is declared dead.

Organ donation

If the patient is suitable for organ donation (Box 12.8), this should be broached with the patient's relatives if it has not been done so

---

Box 12.7. Brain death – testing for apnoea

- Preoxygenate with 100 per cent oxygen for 10 minutes before disconnection
- Allow $PaCO_2$ to rise to 5.0 kPa before the test
- Disconnect from ventilator
- Insufflate oxygen at 6 l/min, via a suction catheter in the trachea, during the period of disconnection
- The $PaCO_2$ must be >6.65 kPa, confirmed by arterial blood gas analysis
- Confirm no respiratory movement
- Reconnect to the ventilator.

Box 12.8. Criteria for organ donation

The potential donor must:

- Be aged 0–75 years
- Have complete and irreversible brainstem damage resulting in brainstem death
- Be maintained on a ventilator
- Have no malignancy (except certain primary brain tumour)
- Have no major systemic sepsis
- Have no social or medical high risk factors for HIV.

---

already. Correct timing is paramount. Ideally, a member of staff who has been appropriately trained and has also built up a rapport with the family should approach relatives. If permission is obtained, the local transplant coordinator should be contacted and the patient managed appropriately.

Management of the organ donor

After consent is obtained for organ donation, optimization of the physiological condition of the donor improves the outcome for organ recipients. However, loss of brainstem function invariably results in pathophysiological changes and complications (Box 12.9), which may make this difficult to achieve. Optimum management requires invasive monitoring. Because of the order in which the great vessels are ligated during a retrieval, the arterial cannula is best located in the left radial or brachial artery and a CVP or pulmonary artery catheter in the right internal jugular vein.

Box 12.9. Incidence of complications after brain death

Hypotension	81 per cent
Diabetes insipidus	65 per cent
Disseminated intravascular coagulation	28 per cent
Cardiac arrhythmias	27 per cent
Pulmonary oedema	18 per cent
Acidosis	11 per cent

Cardiovascular changes

Before complete cessation of brainstem function, medullary ischaemia results in a 'sympathetic storm'. This unopposed sympathetic outflow produces tachycardia, hypertension, arrhythmias and myocardial ischaemia. With brainstem death there is progressive hypotension and bradycardia. ECG abnormalities are common.

- Cardiac output should be optimized using colloid or blood to keep CVP at 10 mmHg
- MAP should be maintained at 70 mmHg
- Dysrhythmias should be treated
- Urinary losses should be replaced with crystalloid
- Inotropic drugs or vasopressors may be used if required.

Pulmonary changes

Hypoxaemia develops, often as a result of pulmonary oedema. Regular physiotherapy and pulmonary suction help to prevent atelectasis and infection. Take care to avoid barotrauma and oxygen toxicity.

Endocrine changes

- Neurogenic diabetes insipidus occurs in up to 70 per cent of individuals. This should be anticipated, as electrolyte abnormalities develop rapidly without treatment (e.g. hypernatraemia, hypokalaemia, hypocalcaemia, hypomagnesaemia and hypophosphataemia). Treatment is with desmopressin (DDAVP) 0.5–4.0 μg boluses, to keep urine output at about 1 mg/kg per hour.
- Pituitary failure causes a fall in circulating tri-iodothyronine (T_3) and thyroxine (T_4), which may contribute to myocardial dysfunction and cardiovascular collapse. Infusions of T_3 3 μg/h may reduce inotropic requirements.

- Insulin secretion is reduced and contributes to the development of hyperglycaemia. Insulin infusions are used to maintain glucose within 6–11 mmol/l.
- Cortisol production is reduced, and boluses of methyl prednisolone 30 mg/kg may be useful in unstable donors.

Renal changes
Renal perfusion may be impaired as a result of the cardiovascular changes mentioned already. Urine output is an important predictor of renal function in the recipient and must be maintained.

Temperature changes
Hypothermia occurs as a result of failure of the thermoregulatory centre in the hypothalamus. The patient should be covered and actively warmed if necessary.

Haematological changes
Haemostatic disorders may occur as a result of tissue thromboplastin releases, and disseminated intravascular coagulation occurs in 28 per cent of donors. Fresh frozen plasma and platelets should be used as necessary.

Index

Lightning Source UK Ltd.
Milton Keynes UK
UKOW052203060212

186767UK00001B/3/A